# www.EffortlessMath.com

## ... So Much More Online!

✓ FREE Math lessons

✓ More Math learning books!

✓ Mathematics Worksheets

✓ Online Math Tutors

**Need a PDF version of this book?**

Please visit www.EffortlessMath.com

# 5 Full-Length DAT Quantitative Reasoning Practice Tests

## *The Practice You Need to Ace the DAT*

## *Quantitative Reasoning Test*

By

Reza Nazari & Ava Ross

All inquiries should be addressed to:

info@effortlessMath.com

www.EffortlessMath.com

**ISBN-13:** 978-1-64612-105-2

**ISBN-10:** 1-64612-105-8

**Published by: Effortless Math Education**

**www.EffortlessMath.com**

# Description

***5 Full-Length DAT Quantitative Reasoning Practice Tests***, which reflects the 2019 and 2020 test guidelines and topics, is designed to help you hone your math skills, overcome your exam anxiety, and boost your confidence -- and do your best to ace the DAT Quantitative Reasoning Test. The realistic and full-length DAT Quantitative Reasoning tests show you how the test is structured and what math topics you need to master. The practice test questions are followed by answer explanations to help you find your weak areas, learn from your mistakes, and raise your DAT Quantitative Reasoning score.

The surest way to succeed on DAT Quantitative Reasoning Test is with intensive practice in every math topic tested-- and that's what you will get in *5 Full-Length DAT Quantitative Reasoning Practice Tests*. This DAT Quantitative Reasoning new edition has been updated to replicate questions appearing on the most recent DAT Quantitative Reasoning tests. This is a precious learning tool for DAT Quantitative Reasoning test takers who need extra practice in math to improve their DAT Quantitative Reasoning score. After taking the DAT Quantitative Reasoning practice tests in this book, you will have solid foundation and adequate practice that is necessary to succeed on the DAT Quantitative Reasoning test. **This book is your ticket to ace the DAT Quantitative Reasoning!**

***5 Full-Length DAT Quantitative Reasoning Practice Tests*** contains many exciting and unique features to help you improve your test scores, including:

- Content 100% aligned with the 2019 - 2020 DAT Quantitative Reasoning test

- Written by DAT Quantitative Reasoning tutors and test experts

- Complete coverage of all DAT Quantitative Reasoning concepts and topics which you will be tested

- Detailed answers and explanations for every DAT Quantitative Reasoning practice questions to help you learn from your mistakes

- 5 full-length practice tests (featuring new question types) with detailed answers

This DAT Quantitative Reasoning book and other Effortless Math Education books are used by thousands of students each year to help them review core content areas, brush-up in math, discover their strengths and weaknesses, and achieve their best scores on the DAT test.

## About the Author

**Reza Nazari** is the author of more than 100 Math learning books including:
– **Math and Critical Thinking Challenges:** For the Middle and High School Student
– **GRE Math in 30 Days**
– **ASVAB Math Workbook 2018 - 2019**
– **Effortless Math Education Workbooks**
– **and many more Mathematics books ...**

Reza is also an experienced Math instructor and a test–prep expert who has been tutoring students since 2008. Reza is the founder of Effortless Math Education, a tutoring company that has helped many students raise their standardized test scores—and attend the colleges of their dreams. Reza provides an individualized custom learning plan and the personalized attention that makes a difference in how students view math.

You can contact Reza via email at:
reza@EffortlessMath.com

Find Reza's professional profile at:
goo.gl/zoC9rJ

# Contents

# DAT Test Review

The Dental Admission Test (also known as the DAT) is a standardized test designed by the American Dental Association (ADA) to measure the general academic skills and perceptual ability of dental school applicants.

The DAT is comprised of multiple-choice test items consisting of four sections:

- ✓ Survey of the Natural Sciences
- ✓ Perceptual Ability
- ✓ Reading Comprehension
- ✓ Quantitative Reasoning

The Quantitative Reasoning section of the DAT measures applicants' math skills that will be required in dental schools. There are 40 multiple-choice questions test takers have 45 minutes to complete this section. A basic four function calculator on the computer screen will be available on this section.

In this book, there are five complete DAT Quantitative Reasoning Tests. Take these tests to see what score you'll be able to receive on a real DAT Quantitative Reasoning test.

Good luck!

# Time to Test

## Time to refine your quantitative reasoning skill with a practice test

Take a DAT Quantitative Reasoning test to simulate the test day experience. After you've finished, score your test using the answer keys.

## Before You Start

- You'll need a pencil, a calculator and a timer to take the test.

- For each question, there are five possible answers. Choose which one is best.

- It's okay to guess. There is no penalty for wrong answers.

- Use the answer sheet provided to record your answers.

- After you've finished the test, review the answer key to see where you went wrong.

**Good Luck!**

# DAT Quantitative Reasoning Practice Test 1

# 2019 - 2020

**Total number of questions:** 40

**Total time:** 45 Minutes

**A basic four function calculator is permitted for DAT Quantitative Reasoning Test.**

# DAT Quantitative Reasoning Practice Tests Answer Sheet

Remove (or photocopy) this answer sheet and use it to complete the practice tests.

## DAT Quantitative Reasoning Practice Test Answer Sheet

DAT Quantitative Reasoning Practice Test 1

| | | | |
|---|---|---|---|
| 1 Ⓐ Ⓑ Ⓒ Ⓓ Ⓔ | 16 Ⓐ Ⓑ Ⓒ Ⓓ Ⓔ | 31 Ⓐ Ⓑ Ⓒ Ⓓ Ⓔ | |
| 2 Ⓐ Ⓑ Ⓒ Ⓓ Ⓔ | 17 Ⓐ Ⓑ Ⓒ Ⓓ Ⓔ | 32 Ⓐ Ⓑ Ⓒ Ⓓ Ⓔ | |
| 3 Ⓐ Ⓑ Ⓒ Ⓓ Ⓔ | 18 Ⓐ Ⓑ Ⓒ Ⓓ Ⓔ | 33 Ⓐ Ⓑ Ⓒ Ⓓ Ⓔ | |
| 4 Ⓐ Ⓑ Ⓒ Ⓓ Ⓔ | 19 Ⓐ Ⓑ Ⓒ Ⓓ Ⓔ | 34 Ⓐ Ⓑ Ⓒ Ⓓ Ⓔ | |
| 5 Ⓐ Ⓑ Ⓒ Ⓓ Ⓔ | 20 Ⓐ Ⓑ Ⓒ Ⓓ Ⓔ | 35 Ⓐ Ⓑ Ⓒ Ⓓ Ⓔ | |
| 6 Ⓐ Ⓑ Ⓒ Ⓓ Ⓔ | 21 Ⓐ Ⓑ Ⓒ Ⓓ Ⓔ | 36 Ⓐ Ⓑ Ⓒ Ⓓ Ⓔ | |
| 7 Ⓐ Ⓑ Ⓒ Ⓓ Ⓔ | 22 Ⓐ Ⓑ Ⓒ Ⓓ Ⓔ | 37 Ⓐ Ⓑ Ⓒ Ⓓ Ⓔ | |
| 8 Ⓐ Ⓑ Ⓒ Ⓓ Ⓔ | 23 Ⓐ Ⓑ Ⓒ Ⓓ Ⓔ | 38 Ⓐ Ⓑ Ⓒ Ⓓ Ⓔ | |
| 9 Ⓐ Ⓑ Ⓒ Ⓓ Ⓔ | 24 Ⓐ Ⓑ Ⓒ Ⓓ Ⓔ | 39 Ⓐ Ⓑ Ⓒ Ⓓ Ⓔ | |
| 10 Ⓐ Ⓑ Ⓒ Ⓓ Ⓔ | 25 Ⓐ Ⓑ Ⓒ Ⓓ Ⓔ | 40 Ⓐ Ⓑ Ⓒ Ⓓ Ⓔ | |
| 11 Ⓐ Ⓑ Ⓒ Ⓓ Ⓔ | 26 Ⓐ Ⓑ Ⓒ Ⓓ Ⓔ | | |
| 12 Ⓐ Ⓑ Ⓒ Ⓓ Ⓔ | 27 Ⓐ Ⓑ Ⓒ Ⓓ Ⓔ | | |
| 13 Ⓐ Ⓑ Ⓒ Ⓓ Ⓔ | 28 Ⓐ Ⓑ Ⓒ Ⓓ Ⓔ | | |
| 14 Ⓐ Ⓑ Ⓒ Ⓓ Ⓔ | 29 Ⓐ Ⓑ Ⓒ Ⓓ Ⓔ | | |
| 15 Ⓐ Ⓑ Ⓒ Ⓓ Ⓔ | 30 Ⓐ Ⓑ Ⓒ Ⓓ Ⓔ | | |

1) In five successive hours, a car traveled $40\ km, 45\ km, 50\ km, 35\ km$ and $55\ km$. In the next five hours, it traveled with an average speed of $65\ km\ per\ hour$. Find the total distance the car traveled in 10 hours.
   A. $425\ km$
   B. $450\ km$
   C. $550\ km$
   D. $600\ km$
   E. $1,000\ km$

2) How long does a 420–miles trip take moving at 65 miles per hour $(mph)$?
   A. $4\ hours$
   B. $6\ hours\ and\ 24\ minutes$
   C. $8\ hours\ and\ 24\ minutes$
   D. $8\ hours\ and\ 30\ minutes$
   E. $10\ hours\ and\ 30\ minutes$

3) Right triangle $ABC$ has two legs of lengths $5\ cm$ $(AB)$ and $12\ cm$ (AC). What is the length of the third side $(BC)$?
   A. $4\ cm$
   B. $6\ cm$
   C. $8\ cm$
   D. $13\ cm$
   E. $20\ cm$

4) The ratio of boys to girls in a school is $2:3$. If there are 500 students in a school, how many boys are in the school?
   A. 540
   B. 360
   C. 300
   D. 280
   E. 200

5) $(7x + 2y)(5x + 2y) = ?$
   A. $2x^2 + 14xy + 2y^2$
   B. $2x^2 + 4xy + 2y^2$
   C. $7x^2 + 14xy + y^2$
   D. $10x^2 + 14xy + 4y$
   E. $35x^2 + 24xy + 4y^2$

6) Which of the following expressions is equivalent to $5x(4 + 2y)$?
   A. $x + 10xy$
   B. $5x + 5xy$
   C. $20xy + 2xy$
   D. $20x + 5xy$
   E. $20x + 10xy$

7) If $y = 5ab + 3b^3$, what is $y$ when $a = 2$ and $b = 3$?
   A. 24
   B. 31
   C. 36
   D. 51
   E. 111

8) 15 is What percent of 20?
   A. 20%
   B. 25%
   C. 75%
   D. 150%
   E. 300%

9) The perimeter of the trapezoid below is 64. What is its area?
   A. $252 \ cm^2$
   B. $234 \ cm^2$
   C. $216 \ cm^2$
   D. $154 \ cm^2$
   E. $260 \ cm^2$

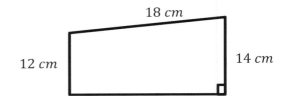

10) Two third of 15 is equal to $\frac{2}{5}$ of what number?
    A. 12
    B. 20
    C. 25
    D. 60
    E. 90

11) The marked price of a computer is $D$ dollar. Its price decreased by 25% in January and later increased by 10% in February. What is the final price of the computer in $D$ dollar?
    A. $0.80 \ D$
    B. $0.82 \ D$
    C. $0.90 \ D$
    D. $1.20 \ D$
    E. $1.40 \ D$

12) The radius of the following cylinder is 8 inches and its height is 14 inches. What is the surface area of the cylinder?

A. $64 \pi \ in^2$
B. $128 \pi \ in^2$
C. $192 \pi in^2$
D. $256 \pi \ in^2$
E. $352 \pi in^2$

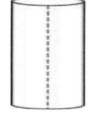

13) The average of $13, 15, 20$ and $x$ is $20$. What is the value of $x$?

A. 9
B. 15
C. 18
D. 20
E. 32

14) The price of a sofa is decreased by 25% to $450. What was its original price?

A. $480
B. $520
C. $560
D. $600
E. $800

15) The area of a circle is $49 \pi$. What is the circumference of the circle?

A. $7 \pi$
B. $14 \pi$
C. $32 \pi$
D. $64 \pi$
E. $124 \pi$

16) A $50 shirt now selling for $28 is discounted by what percent?

A. 20%
B. 44%
C. 54%
D. 60%
E. 80%

17) In 1999, the average worker's income increased $2,000 per year starting from $26,000 annual salary. Which equation represents income greater than average? ($I$ = income, $x$ = number of years after 1999)

A. $I > 2000 \, x + 26000$
B. $I > -2000 \, x + 26000$
C. $I < -2000 \, x + 26000$
D. $I < 2000 \, x - 26000$
E. $I < 24,000 \, x + 26000$

18) A boat sails 60 miles south and then 80 miles east. How far is the boat from its start point?
    A. 45 *miles*
    B. 50 *miles*
    C. 60 *miles*
    D. 70 *miles*
    E. 100 *miles*

19) Sophia purchased a sofa for $530.40. The sofa is regularly priced at $631. What was the percent discount Sophia received on the sofa?
    A. 12%
    B. 16%
    C. 20%
    D. 25%
    E. 40%

20) The score of Emma was half as that of Ava and the score of Mia was twice that of Ava. If the score of Mia was 40, what is the score of Emma?
    A. 10
    B. 15
    C. 20
    D. 30
    E. 40

21) A bag contains 18 balls: two green, five black, eight blue, a brown, a red and one white. If 17 balls are removed from the bag at random, what is the probability that a brown ball has been removed?
    A. $\frac{1}{9}$
    B. $\frac{1}{6}$
    C. $\frac{16}{11}$
    D. $\frac{17}{18}$
    E. $\frac{1}{2}$

22) The average of five consecutive numbers is 36. What is the smallest number?
    A. 38
    B. 36
    C. 34
    D. 12
    E. 8

23) The price of a car was $28,000 in 2012. In 2013, the price of that car was $18,200. What was the rate of depreciation of the price of car per year?
   A. 20%
   B. 30%
   C. 35%
   D. 40%
   E. 50%

24) The width of a box is one third of its length. The height of the box is one third of its width. If the length of the box is 36 $cm$, what is the volume of the box?
   A. 81 $cm^3$
   B. 162 $cm^3$
   C. 243 $cm^3$
   D. 1,728 $cm^3$
   E. 1,880 $cm^3$

25) A tree 32 feet tall casts a shadow 12 feet long. Jack is 6 feet tall. How long is Jack's shadow?
   A. 2.25 $feet$
   B. 4 $feet$
   C. 4.25 $feet$
   D. 8 $feet$
   E. 12 $feet$

26) When a number is subtracted from 28 and the difference is divided by that number, the result is 3. What is the value of the number?
   A. 2
   B. 4
   C. 7
   D. 12
   E. 24

27) An angle is equal to one ninth of its supplement. What is the measure of that angle?
   A. 9
   B. 18
   C. 25
   D. 60
   E. 90

28) John traveled 150 $km$ in 6 hours and Alice traveled 140 $km$ in 4 hours. What is the ratio of the average speed of John to average speed of Alice?
   A. 3 : 2
   B. 2 : 3
   C. 5 : 7
   D. 5 : 6
   E. 11 : 16

29) If 45% of a class are girls, and 25% of girls play tennis, what percent of the class play tennis?
   A. 11%
   B. 15%
   C. 20%
   D. 40%
   E. 80%

30) How many tiles of 8 $cm^2$ is needed to cover a floor of dimension 7 $cm$ by 24 $cm$?
   A. 6
   B. 12
   C. 18
   D. 21
   E. 36

31) A rope weighs 600 grams per meter of length. What is the weight in kilograms of 14.2 meters of this rope? (1 $kilograms = 1,000\ grams$)
   A. 0.0852
   B. 0.852
   C. 8.52
   D. 8,520
   E. 85,200

32) A chemical solution contains 6% alcohol. If there is 24 $ml$ of alcohol, what is the volume of the solution?
   A. 240 $ml$
   B. 400 $ml$
   C. 600 $ml$
   D. 1,200 $ml$
   E. 2,400 $ml$

33) The average weight of 18 girls in a class is 56 $kg$ and the average weight of 32 boys in the same class is 62 $kg$. What is the average weight of all the 50 students in that class?
   A. 50
   B. 59.84
   C. 61.68
   D. 61.90
   E. 62.20

34) The price of a laptop is decreased by 20% to $360. What is its original price?
   A. $320
   B. $380
   C. $400
   D. $450
   E. $500

35) A bank is offering 4.5% simple interest on a savings account. If you deposit $9,000, how much interest will you earn in five years?

A. $360

B. $720

C. $2,025

D. $3,600

E. $4,800

36) Multiply and write the product in scientific notation:
$$(2.9 \times 10^6) \times (2.6 \times 10^{-5})$$

A. $754 \times 100$

B. $75.4 \times 10^6$

C. $75.4 \times 10^{-5}$

D. $7.54 \times 10^{11}$

E. $7.54 \times 10$

37) If the height of a right pyramid is $14\ cm$ and its base is a square with side $6\ cm$. What is its volume?

A. $432\ cm^3$

B. $3088\ cm^3$

C. $236\ cm^3$

D. $172\ cm^3$

E. $168\ cm^3$

38) 5 less than twice a positive integer is 73. What is the integer?

A. 39

B. 41

C. 42

D. 44

E. 50

39) A shirt costing $300 is discounted 15%. After a month, the shirt is discounted another 15%. Which of the following expressions can be used to find the selling price of the shirt?

A. $(300)\,(0.70)$

B. $(300) - 300\,(0.30)$

C. $(300)(0.15) - (300)\,(0.15)$

D. $(300)\,(0.85)(0.85)$

E. $(300)(0.85)(0.85) - (300)\,(0.15)$

40) Which of the following points lies on the line $2x + 4y = 8$?
   A. $(2, 1)$
   B. $(-1, 3)$
   C. $(-2, 2)$
   D. $(2, 2)$
   E. $(2, 8)$

## End of DAT Quantitative Reasoning Practice Test 1

# DAT Quantitative Reasoning Practice Test 2

## 2019 - 2020

**Total number of questions:** 40

**Total time:** 45 Minutes

**A basic four function calculator is permitted for DAT Quantitative Reasoning Test.**

# DAT Quantitative Reasoning Practice Tests Answer Sheet

**Remove (or photocopy) this answer sheet and use it to complete the practice tests.**

**DAT Quantitative Reasoning Practice Test Answer Sheet**

DAT Quantitative Reasoning Practice Test 2

| # | | # | | # | |
|---|---|---|---|---|---|
| 1 | (A) (B) (C) (D) (E) | 16 | (A) (B) (C) (D) (E) | 31 | (A) (B) (C) (D) (E) |
| 2 | (A) (B) (C) (D) (E) | 17 | (A) (B) (C) (D) (E) | 32 | (A) (B) (C) (D) (E) |
| 3 | (A) (B) (C) (D) (E) | 18 | (A) (B) (C) (D) (E) | 33 | (A) (B) (C) (D) (E) |
| 4 | (A) (B) (C) (D) (E) | 19 | (A) (B) (C) (D) (E) | 34 | (A) (B) (C) (D) (E) |
| 5 | (A) (B) (C) (D) (E) | 20 | (A) (B) (C) (D) (E) | 35 | (A) (B) (C) (D) (E) |
| 6 | (A) (B) (C) (D) (E) | 21 | (A) (B) (C) (D) (E) | 36 | (A) (B) (C) (D) (E) |
| 7 | (A) (B) (C) (D) (E) | 22 | (A) (B) (C) (D) (E) | 37 | (A) (B) (C) (D) (E) |
| 8 | (A) (B) (C) (D) (E) | 23 | (A) (B) (C) (D) (E) | 38 | (A) (B) (C) (D) (E) |
| 9 | (A) (B) (C) (D) (E) | 24 | (A) (B) (C) (D) (E) | 39 | (A) (B) (C) (D) (E) |
| 10 | (A) (B) (C) (D) (E) | 25 | (A) (B) (C) (D) (E) | 40 | (A) (B) (C) (D) (E) |
| 11 | (A) (B) (C) (D) (E) | 26 | (A) (B) (C) (D) (E) | | |
| 12 | (A) (B) (C) (D) (E) | 27 | (A) (B) (C) (D) (E) | | |
| 13 | (A) (B) (C) (D) (E) | 28 | (A) (B) (C) (D) (E) | | |
| 14 | (A) (B) (C) (D) (E) | 29 | (A) (B) (C) (D) (E) | | |
| 15 | (A) (B) (C) (D) (E) | 30 | (A) (B) (C) (D) (E) | | |

1) The mean of 50 test scores was calculated as 90. But, it turned out that one of the scores was misread as 94 but it was 69. What is the mean?
   A. 85
   B. 87
   C. 89.5
   D. 90.5
   E. 95.5

2) Two dice are thrown simultaneously, what is the probability of getting a sum of 5 or 8?
   A. $\frac{1}{3}$
   B. $\frac{11}{36}$
   C. $\frac{1}{16}$
   D. $\frac{1}{4}$
   E. $\frac{1}{36}$

3) Which of the following is equal to the expression below?

$$(5x + 2y)(2x - y)$$

   A. $4x^2 - 2y^2$
   B. $2x^2 + 6xy - 2y^2$
   C. $24x^2 + 2xy - 2y^2$
   D. $10x^2 - xy - 2y^2$
   E. $8x^2 + 2xy - 2y^2$

4) What is the product of all possible values of $x$ in the following equation?

$$|x - 10| = 4$$

   A. 3
   B. 7
   C. 13
   D. 84
   E. 100

5) What is the slope of a line that is perpendicular to the line
$$4x - 2y = 6?$$
   A. $-2$
   B. $-\frac{1}{2}$
   C. 4
   D. 12
   E. 14

6) What is the value of the expression $6(x - 2y) + (2 - x)^2$ when $x = 3$ and $= -2$ ?
   A.  $-4$
   B.  20
   C.  43
   D.  50
   E.  80

7) A swimming pool holds 2,500 cubic feet of water. The swimming pool is 25 feet long and 10 feet wide. How deep is the swimming pool?
   A.  $2\ feet$
   B.  $4\ feet$
   C.  $6\ feet$
   D.  $7\ feet$
   E.  $10\ feet$

8) Four one – foot rulers can be split among how many users to leave each with $\frac{1}{3}$ of a ruler?
   A.  4
   B.  6
   C.  12
   D.  24
   E.  48

9) What is the area of a square whose diagonal is 4?
   A.  4
   B.  8
   C.  16
   D.  64
   E.  124

10) The average of five numbers is 26. If a sixth number 42 is added, then, what is the new average? (round your answer to the nearest hundredth)
   A.  25
   B.  26.5
   C.  27
   D.  28.66
   E.  36

11) The ratio of boys and girls in a class is 4: 7. If there are 55 students in the class, how many more boys should be enrolled to make the ratio 1: 1?
   A.  8
   B.  10
   C.  15
   D.  20
   E.  28

12) Mr. Jones saves $2,500 out of his monthly family income of $65,000. What fractional part of his income does he save?
   A.  $\frac{1}{26}$
   B.  $\frac{1}{11}$
   C.  $\frac{3}{25}$
   D.  $\frac{2}{15}$
   E.  $\frac{1}{15}$

13) A football team had $20,000 to spend on supplies. The team spent $14,000 on new balls. New sport shoes cost $110 each. Which of the following inequalities represent how many new shoes the team can purchase.
   A.  $110x + 14,000 \le 20,000$
   B.  $110x + 14,000 \ge 20,000$
   C.  $14,000x + 110 \le 20,000$
   D.  $14,000x + 110 \ge 20,000$
   E.  $14,000x + 14000 \ge 20,000$

14) Jason needs an 70% average in his writing class to pass. On his first 4 exams, he earned scores of 68%, 72%, 85%, and 90%. What is the minimum score Jason can earn on his fifth and final test to pass?
   A.  80%,
   B.  70%
   C.  68%
   D.  54%
   E.  35%

15) What is the value of $x$ in the following equation?

$$\frac{2}{3}x + \frac{1}{6} = \frac{1}{2}$$

A. 6

B. $\frac{1}{2}$

C. $\frac{1}{3}$

D. $\frac{1}{4}$

E. $\frac{1}{12}$

16) A bank is offering 4.5% simple interest on a savings account. If you deposit $12,000, how much interest will you earn in two years?
A. $420
B. $1,080
C. $4,200
D. $8,400
E. $9,600

17) Simplify $7x^2y^3(2x^2y)^3 =$

A. $12x^4y^6$
B. $12x^8y^6$
C. $56x^4y^6$
D. $56x^8y^6$
E. $96x^8y^6$

18) What is the surface area of the cylinder below?

A. $40\,\pi\,in^2$
B. $57\,\pi\,in^2$
C. $66\,\pi\,in^2$
D. $288\,\pi\,in^2$
E. $400\,\pi\,in^2$

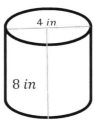

4 in

8 in

19) Last week 25,000 fans attended a football match. This week three times as many bought tickets, but one sixth of them cancelled their tickets. How many are attending this week?
A. 48,000
B. 54,000
C. 62,500
D. 75,000
E. 84,000

20) What is the perimeter of a square that has an area of 49 square inches?
   A. $144\ inches$
   B. $64\ inches$
   C. $56\ inches$
   D. $48\ inches$
   E. $28\ inches$

21) If $f(x)=2x^3+5x^2+2x$ and $g(x)=-4$, what is the value of $f(g(x))$?

   A. 56
   B. 32
   C. 24
   D. $-4$
   E. $-56$

22) A cruise line ship left Port A and traveled 50 miles due west and then 120 miles due north. At this point, what is the shortest distance from the cruise to port A?
   A. $70\ miles$
   B. $80\ miles$
   C. $150\ miles$
   D. $230\ miles$
   E. $130\ miles$

23) What is the equivalent temperature of $104°F$ in Celsius?
   $$C = \frac{5}{9}(F-32)$$
   A. 32
   B. 40
   C. 48
   D. 52
   E. 64

24) The perimeter of a rectangular yard is 72 meters. What is its length if its width is twice its length?
   A. $12\ meters$
   B. $18\ meters$
   C. $20\ meters$
   D. $24\ meters$
   E. $36\ meters$

25) The average of 6 numbers is 14. The average of 4 of those numbers is 10. What is the average of the other two numbers?
   A. 10
   B. 12
   C. 14
   D. 22
   E. 24

26) If 150% of a number is 75, then what is the 80% of that number?
   A. 40
   B. 50
   C. 70
   D. 85
   E. 90

27) What is the slope of the line: $4x - 2y = 12$
   A. $-1$
   B. $-2$
   C. 1
   D. 1.5
   E. 2

28) In two successive years, the population of a town is increased by 10% and 20%. What percent of the population is increased after two years?
   A. 30%
   B. 32%
   C. 35%
   D. 68%
   E. 70%

29) The area of a circle is $36\pi$. What is the diameter of the circle?
   A. 4
   B. 8
   C. 12
   D. 14
   E. 16

30) If 20% of a number is 4, what is the number?
   A. 4
   B. 8
   C. 10
   D. 20
   E. 25

31) If a tree casts a 26–foot shadow at the same time that a 3 feet yardstick casts a 2–foot shadow, what is the height of the tree?

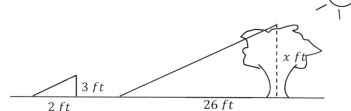

A. 24 *ft*
B. 28 *ft*
C. 39 *ft*
D. 48 *ft*
E. 52 *ft*

32) Jason is 9 miles ahead of Joe running at 6.5 miles per hour and Joe is running at the speed of 8 miles per hour. How long does it take Joe to catch Jason?

A. 3 *hours*
B. 4 *hours*
C. 6 *hours*
D. 8 *hours*
E. 10 *hours*

33) 44 students took an exam and 11 of them failed. What percent of the students passed the exam?

A. 20%
B. 40%
C. 60%
D. 75%
E. 90%

34) If $f(x) = 2x^3 + 5x^2 + 2x$ and $g(x) = -3$, what is the value of $f(g(x))$?

A. 36
B. 32
C. 24
D. 15
E. −15

35) The diagonal of a rectangle is 10 inches long and the height of the rectangle is 6 inches. What is the perimeter of the rectangle?

A. 10 *inches*
B. 12 *inches*
C. 16 *inches*
D. 18 *inches*
E. 28 *inches*

36) The perimeter of the trapezoid below is 40 $cm$. What is its area?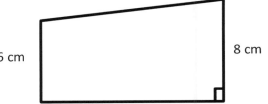

    A. 48 $cm^2$
    B. 98 $cm^2$
    C. 140 $cm^2$
    D. 576 $cm^2$
    E. 986 $cm^2$

37) If $f(x)=2x^3+2$ and $(x)=\frac{1}{x}$, what is the value of $f(g(x))$?

    A. $\dfrac{1}{2x^3+2}$

    B. $\dfrac{2}{x^3}$

    C. $\dfrac{1}{2x}$

    D. $\dfrac{1}{2x+2}$

    E. $\dfrac{2}{x^3}+2$

38) A cruise line ship left Port $A$ and traveled 80 miles due west and then 150 miles due north.

    At this point, what is the shortest distance from the cruise to port $A$?

    A. 70 miles

    B. 80 miles

    C. 150 miles

    D. 170 miles

    E. 230 miles

39) If the ratio of $5a$ to $2b$ is $\frac{1}{10}$, what is the ratio of $a$ to $b$?

    A. 10

    B. 25

    C. $\dfrac{1}{25}$

    D. $\dfrac{1}{20}$

    E. $\dfrac{1}{10}$

40) If $x = 9$, what is the value of $y$ in the following equation?

$$2y = \frac{2x^2}{3} + 6$$

A. 30

B. 45

C. 60

D. 120

E. 180

**End of DAT Quantitative Reasoning Practice Test 2**

# DAT Quantitative Reasoning Practice Test 3

## 2019 - 2020

**Total number of questions:** 40

**Total time:** 45 Minutes

**A basic four function calculator is permitted for DAT Quantitative Reasoning Test.**

# DAT Quantitative Reasoning Practice Tests Answer Sheet

Remove (or photocopy) this answer sheet and use it to complete the practice tests.

## DAT Quantitative Reasoning Practice Test Answer Sheet

DAT Quantitative Reasoning Practice Test 3

| | | | |
|---|---|---|---|
| 1 Ⓐ Ⓑ Ⓒ Ⓓ Ⓔ | 16 Ⓐ Ⓑ Ⓒ Ⓓ Ⓔ | 31 Ⓐ Ⓑ Ⓒ Ⓓ Ⓔ | Ⓐ Ⓑ Ⓒ Ⓓ Ⓔ |
| 2 Ⓐ Ⓑ Ⓒ Ⓓ Ⓔ | 17 Ⓐ Ⓑ Ⓒ Ⓓ Ⓔ | 32 Ⓐ Ⓑ Ⓒ Ⓓ Ⓔ | Ⓐ Ⓑ Ⓒ Ⓓ Ⓔ |
| 3 Ⓐ Ⓑ Ⓒ Ⓓ Ⓔ | 18 Ⓐ Ⓑ Ⓒ Ⓓ Ⓔ | 33 Ⓐ Ⓑ Ⓒ Ⓓ Ⓔ | Ⓐ Ⓑ Ⓒ Ⓓ Ⓔ |
| 4 Ⓐ Ⓑ Ⓒ Ⓓ Ⓔ | 19 Ⓐ Ⓑ Ⓒ Ⓓ Ⓔ | 34 Ⓐ Ⓑ Ⓒ Ⓓ Ⓔ | Ⓐ Ⓑ Ⓒ Ⓓ Ⓔ |
| 5 Ⓐ Ⓑ Ⓒ Ⓓ Ⓔ | 20 Ⓐ Ⓑ Ⓒ Ⓓ Ⓔ | 35 Ⓐ Ⓑ Ⓒ Ⓓ Ⓔ | Ⓐ Ⓑ Ⓒ Ⓓ Ⓔ |
| 6 Ⓐ Ⓑ Ⓒ Ⓓ Ⓔ | 21 Ⓐ Ⓑ Ⓒ Ⓓ Ⓔ | 36 Ⓐ Ⓑ Ⓒ Ⓓ Ⓔ | Ⓐ Ⓑ Ⓒ Ⓓ Ⓔ |
| 7 Ⓐ Ⓑ Ⓒ Ⓓ Ⓔ | 22 Ⓐ Ⓑ Ⓒ Ⓓ Ⓔ | 37 Ⓐ Ⓑ Ⓒ Ⓓ Ⓔ | Ⓐ Ⓑ Ⓒ Ⓓ Ⓔ |
| 8 Ⓐ Ⓑ Ⓒ Ⓓ Ⓔ | 23 Ⓐ Ⓑ Ⓒ Ⓓ Ⓔ | 38 Ⓐ Ⓑ Ⓒ Ⓓ Ⓔ | Ⓐ Ⓑ Ⓒ Ⓓ Ⓔ |
| 9 Ⓐ Ⓑ Ⓒ Ⓓ Ⓔ | 24 Ⓐ Ⓑ Ⓒ Ⓓ Ⓔ | 39 Ⓐ Ⓑ Ⓒ Ⓓ Ⓔ | Ⓐ Ⓑ Ⓒ Ⓓ Ⓔ |
| 10 Ⓐ Ⓑ Ⓒ Ⓓ Ⓔ | 25 Ⓐ Ⓑ Ⓒ Ⓓ Ⓔ | 40 Ⓐ Ⓑ Ⓒ Ⓓ Ⓔ | Ⓐ Ⓑ Ⓒ Ⓓ Ⓔ |
| 11 Ⓐ Ⓑ Ⓒ Ⓓ Ⓔ | 26 Ⓐ Ⓑ Ⓒ Ⓓ Ⓔ | | |
| 12 Ⓐ Ⓑ Ⓒ Ⓓ Ⓔ | 27 Ⓐ Ⓑ Ⓒ Ⓓ Ⓔ | | |
| 13 Ⓐ Ⓑ Ⓒ Ⓓ Ⓔ | 28 Ⓐ Ⓑ Ⓒ Ⓓ Ⓔ | | |
| 14 Ⓐ Ⓑ Ⓒ Ⓓ Ⓔ | 29 Ⓐ Ⓑ Ⓒ Ⓓ Ⓔ | | |
| 15 Ⓐ Ⓑ Ⓒ Ⓓ Ⓔ | 30 Ⓐ Ⓑ Ⓒ Ⓓ Ⓔ | | |

1) When a number is subtracted from 24 and the difference is divided by that number, the result is 3. What is the value of the number?
   A. 2
   B. 4
   C. 6
   D. 12
   E. 24

2) An angle is equal to one fifth of its supplement. What is the measure of that angle?
   A. 20
   B. 30
   C. 45
   D. 60
   E. 90

3) John traveled 150 $km$ in 6 hours and Alice traveled 180 $km$ in 4 hours. What is the ratio of the average speed of John to average speed of Alice?
   A. $3 : 2$
   B. $2 : 3$
   C. $5 : 9$
   D. $5 : 6$
   E. $11 : 16$

4) If 40% of a class are girls, and 35% of girls play tennis, what percent of the class play tennis?
   A. 10%
   B. 14%
   C. 20%
   D. 40%
   E. 80%

5) In five successive hours, a car traveled 40 $km$, 45 $km$, 50 $km$, 35 $km$ and 55 $km$. In the next five hours, it traveled with an average speed of 50 $km\ per\ hour$. Find the total distance the car traveled in 10 hours.
   A. 425 $km$
   B. 450 $km$
   C. 475 $km$
   D. 500 $km$
   E. 1,000 $km$

6) How long does a 420–miles trip take moving at 50 miles per hour ($mph$)?
   A. 4 *hours*
   B. 6 *hours and* 24 *minutes*
   C. 8 *hours and* 24 *minutes*
   D. 8 *hours and* 30 *minutes*
   E. 10 *hours and* 30 *minutes*

7) Right triangle $ABC$ has two legs of lengths 6 $cm$ ($AB$) and 8 $cm$ ($AC$). What is the length of the third side ($BC$)?
   A. 4 $cm$
   B. 6 $cm$
   C. 8 $cm$
   D. 10 $cm$
   E. 20 $cm$

8) The ratio of boys to girls in a school is 2: 3. If there are 600 students in a school, how many boys are in the school.
   A. 540
   B. 360
   C. 300
   D. 280
   E. 240

9) 25 is What percent of 20?
   A. 20%
   B. 25%
   C. 125%
   D. 150%
   E. 300%

10) The perimeter of the trapezoid below is 54. What is its area?
   A. 252 $cm^2$
   B. 234 $cm^2$
   C. 216 $cm^2$
   D. 154 $cm^2$
   E. 130$cm^2$

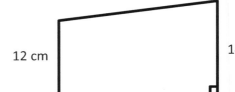

18 cm

12 cm

14 cm

11) Two third of 18 is equal to $\frac{2}{5}$ of what number?

   A. 12
   B. 20
   C. 30
   D. 60
   E. 90

12) The marked price of a computer is $D$ dollar. Its price decreased by 20% in January and later increased by 10% in February. What is the final price of the computer in $D$ dollar?

   A. 0.80 $D$
   B. 0.88 $D$
   C. 0.90 $D$
   D. 1.20 $D$
   E. 1.40 $D$

13) The area of a circle is 25 $\pi$. What is the circumference of the circle?

   A. 5 $\pi$
   B. 10 $\pi$
   C. 32 $\pi$
   D. 64 $\pi$
   E. 124 $\pi$

14) In 1999, the average worker's income increased $3,000 per year starting from $24,000 annual salary. Which equation represents income greater than average? ($I$ = income, $x$ = number of years after 1999)

   A. $I > 3000\, x + 24000$
   B. $I > -3000\, x + 24000$
   C. $I < -3000\, x + 24000$
   D. $I < 3000\, x - 24000$
   E. $I < 24,000\, x + 24000$

15) From last year, the price of gasoline has increased from $1.25 per gallon to $1.75 per gallon. The new price is what percent of the original price?

   A. 72%
   B. 120%
   C. 140%
   D. 160%
   E. 180%

16) A boat sails 40 miles south and then 30 miles east. How far is the boat from its start point?
   A. 45 $miles$
   B. 50 $miles$
   C. 60 $miles$
   D. 70 $miles$
   E. 80 $miles$

17) Sophia purchased a sofa for $530.40. The sofa is regularly priced at $624. What was the percent discount Sophia received on the sofa?
   A. 12%
   B. 15%
   C. 20%
   D. 25%
   E. 40%

18) The score of Emma was half as that of Ava and the score of Mia was twice that of Ava. If the score of Mia was 60, what is the score of Emma?
   A. 12
   B. 15
   C. 20
   D. 30
   E. 40

19) The average of five consecutive numbers is 38. What is the smallest number?
   A. 38
   B. 36
   C. 34
   D. 12
   E. 8

20) How many tiles of 8 $cm^2$ is needed to cover a floor of dimension 6 $cm$ by 24 $cm$?
   A. 6
   B. 12
   C. 18
   D. 24

   E. 36
21) A rope weighs 600 grams per meter of length. What is the weight in kilograms of 12.2 meters of this rope? (1 $kilograms$ = 1000 $grams$)
   A. 0.0732
   B. 0.732
   C. 7.32
   D. 7,320
   E. 73,200

22) A chemical solution contains 4% alcohol. If there is 24 $ml$ of alcohol, what is the volume of the solution?
    A. 240 $ml$
    B. 480 $ml$
    C. 600 $ml$
    D. 1,200 $ml$
    E. 2,400 $ml$

23) The average weight of 18 girls in a class is 60 $kg$ and the average weight of 32 boys in the same class is 62 $kg$. What is the average weight of all the 50 students in that class?
    A. 60
    B. 61.28
    C. 61.68
    D. 61.90
    E. 62.20

24) The price of a laptop is decreased by 10% to $360. What is its original price?
    A. $320
    B. $380
    C. $400
    D. $450
    E. $500

25) The radius of the following cylinder is 8 inches and its height is 12 inches. What is the surface area of the cylinder?
    A. 64 $\pi$ $in^2$
    B. 128 $\pi$ $in^2$
    C. 192 $\pi$ $in^2$
    D. 256 $\pi$ $in^2$
    E. 320 $\pi$ $in^2$

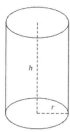

26) The average of 13, 15, 20 and $x$ is 18. What is the value of $x$?
    A. 9
    B. 15
    C. 18
    D. 20
    E. 24

27) The price of a sofa is decreased by 25% to $420. What was its original price?
    A. $480
    B. $520
    C. $560
    D. $600
    E. $800

28) A bank is offering 4.5% simple interest on a savings account. If you deposit $8,000, how much interest will you earn in five years?
   A. $360
   B. $720
   C. $1,800
   D. $3,600
   E. $4,800

29) Multiply and write the product in scientific notation:

$$(4.2 \times 10^6) \times (2.6 \times 10^{-5})$$

   A. $1092 \times 10$
   B. $10.92 \times 10^6$
   C. $109.2 \times 10^{-5}$
   D. $10.92 \times 10^{11}$
   E. $1.092 \times 10^2$

30) If the height of a right pyramid is $12\ cm$ and its base is a square with side $6\ cm$. What is its volume?
   A. $32\ cm^3$
   B. $36\ cm^3$
   C. $48\ cm^3$
   D. $72\ cm^3$
   E. $144\ cm^3$

31) Solve for $x$: $4(x + 1) = 6(x - 4) + 20$
   A. 12
   B. 8
   C. 6.2
   D. 5.5
   E. 4

32) Which of the following expressions is equivalent to

$$2x\,(4 + 2y)?$$

   A. $2xy + 8x$
   B. $8xy + 8x$
   C. $xy + 8$
   D. $2xy + 8x$
   E. $4xy + 8x$

33) If $y = 4ab + 3b^3$, what is y when $a = 2$ and $b = 3$?
   A. 24
   B. 31
   C. 36
   D. 51
   E. 105

34) 11 yards 6 feet and 4 inches equals to how many inches?
   A. 388
   B. 468
   C. 472
   D. 476
   E. 486

35) 5 less than twice a positive integer is 83. What is the integer?
   A. 39
   B. 41
   C. 42
   D. 44
   E. 50

36) A shirt costing $200 is discounted 15%. After a month, the shirt is discounted another 15%. Which of the following expressions can be used to find the selling price of the shirt?
   A. $(200)(0.70)$
   B. $(200) - 200(0.30)$
   C. $(200)(0.15) - (200)(0.15)$
   D. $(200)(0.85)(0.85)$
   E. $(200)(0.85)(0.85) - (200)(0.15)$

37) Which of the following points lies on the line $2x + 4y = 10$
   A. $(2, 1)$
   B. $(-1, 3)$
   C. $(-2, 2)$
   D. $(2, 2)$
   E. $(2, 8)$

38) The price of a car was $20,000 in 2014, $16,000 in 2015 and $12,800 in 2016. What is the rate of depreciation of the price of car per year?
   A. 15%
   B. 20%
   C. 25%
   D. 30%
   E. 50%

39) A ladder leans against a wall forming a 60° angle between the ground and the ladder. If the bottom of the ladder is 30 feet away from the wall, how long is the ladder?

A. $30\ feet$

B. $40\ feet$

C. $50\ feet$

D. $60\ feet$

E. $120\ feet$

40) Right triangle $ABC$ is shown below. Which of the following is true for all possible values of angle $A$ and $B$?

A. $\tan A = \tan B$

B. $\sin A = \cos B$

C. $\tan^2 A = \tan^2 B$

D. $\tan A = 1$

E. $\cot A = \sin B$

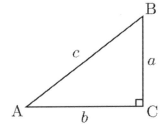

# End of DAT Quantitative Reasoning Practice Test 3

# DAT Quantitative Reasoning Practice Test 4

## 2019 - 2020

**Total number of questions:** 40

**Total time:** 45 Minutes

**A basic four function calculator is permitted for DAT Quantitative Reasoning Test.**

# DAT Quantitative Reasoning Practice Tests Answer Sheet

Remove (or photocopy) this answer sheet and use it to complete the practice tests.

### DAT Quantitative Reasoning Practice Test Answer Sheet

DAT Quantitative Reasoning Practice Test 4

| | | | |
|---|---|---|---|
| 1 | Ⓐ Ⓑ Ⓒ Ⓓ Ⓔ | 16 | Ⓐ Ⓑ Ⓒ Ⓓ Ⓔ | 31 | Ⓐ Ⓑ Ⓒ Ⓓ Ⓔ |
| 2 | Ⓐ Ⓑ Ⓒ Ⓓ Ⓔ | 17 | Ⓐ Ⓑ Ⓒ Ⓓ Ⓔ | 32 | Ⓐ Ⓑ Ⓒ Ⓓ Ⓔ |
| 3 | Ⓐ Ⓑ Ⓒ Ⓓ Ⓔ | 18 | Ⓐ Ⓑ Ⓒ Ⓓ Ⓔ | 33 | Ⓐ Ⓑ Ⓒ Ⓓ Ⓔ |
| 4 | Ⓐ Ⓑ Ⓒ Ⓓ Ⓔ | 19 | Ⓐ Ⓑ Ⓒ Ⓓ Ⓔ | 34 | Ⓐ Ⓑ Ⓒ Ⓓ Ⓔ |
| 5 | Ⓐ Ⓑ Ⓒ Ⓓ Ⓔ | 20 | Ⓐ Ⓑ Ⓒ Ⓓ Ⓔ | 35 | Ⓐ Ⓑ Ⓒ Ⓓ Ⓔ |
| 6 | Ⓐ Ⓑ Ⓒ Ⓓ Ⓔ | 21 | Ⓐ Ⓑ Ⓒ Ⓓ Ⓔ | 36 | Ⓐ Ⓑ Ⓒ Ⓓ Ⓔ |
| 7 | Ⓐ Ⓑ Ⓒ Ⓓ Ⓔ | 22 | Ⓐ Ⓑ Ⓒ Ⓓ Ⓔ | 37 | Ⓐ Ⓑ Ⓒ Ⓓ Ⓔ |
| 8 | Ⓐ Ⓑ Ⓒ Ⓓ Ⓔ | 23 | Ⓐ Ⓑ Ⓒ Ⓓ Ⓔ | 38 | Ⓐ Ⓑ Ⓒ Ⓓ Ⓔ |
| 9 | Ⓐ Ⓑ Ⓒ Ⓓ Ⓔ | 24 | Ⓐ Ⓑ Ⓒ Ⓓ Ⓔ | 39 | Ⓐ Ⓑ Ⓒ Ⓓ Ⓔ |
| 10 | Ⓐ Ⓑ Ⓒ Ⓓ Ⓔ | 25 | Ⓐ Ⓑ Ⓒ Ⓓ Ⓔ | 40 | Ⓐ Ⓑ Ⓒ Ⓓ Ⓔ |
| 11 | Ⓐ Ⓑ Ⓒ Ⓓ Ⓔ | 26 | Ⓐ Ⓑ Ⓒ Ⓓ Ⓔ | | |
| 12 | Ⓐ Ⓑ Ⓒ Ⓓ Ⓔ | 27 | Ⓐ Ⓑ Ⓒ Ⓓ Ⓔ | | |
| 13 | Ⓐ Ⓑ Ⓒ Ⓓ Ⓔ | 28 | Ⓐ Ⓑ Ⓒ Ⓓ Ⓔ | | |
| 14 | Ⓐ Ⓑ Ⓒ Ⓓ Ⓔ | 29 | Ⓐ Ⓑ Ⓒ Ⓓ Ⓔ | | |
| 15 | Ⓐ Ⓑ Ⓒ Ⓓ Ⓔ | 30 | Ⓐ Ⓑ Ⓒ Ⓓ Ⓔ | | |

1) If $f(x) = 3x^3 + 5x^2 + 2x$ and $g(x) = -2$, what is the value of $f(g(x))$?
   A. 36
   B. 32
   C. 24
   D. 8
   E. $-8$

2) The diagonal of a rectangle is 10 inches long and the height of the rectangle is 8 inches. What is the perimeter of the rectangle?
   A. 10 *inches*
   B. 12 *inches*
   C. 16 *inches*
   D. 18 *inches*
   E. 28 *inches*

3) If $x = \frac{1}{3}$ and $y = \frac{9}{21}$, then which is equal to $\frac{1}{x} \div \frac{y}{3}$?
   A. $\frac{1}{7}$
   B. $\frac{1}{21}$
   C. $\frac{1}{3}$
   D. 9
   E. 21

4) The mean of 50 test scores was calculated as 85. But, it turned out that one of the scores was misread as 94 but it was 69. What is the mean?
   A. 84.5
   B. 87
   C. 87.5
   D. 88.5
   E. 90.5

5) Which of the following answers represents the compound inequality $-4 \leq 4x - 8 < 16$?
   A. $-2 \leq x \leq 8$
   B. $-2 < x \leq 8$
   C. $1 < x \leq 6$
   D. $1 \leq x < 6$
   E. $2 \leq x \leq 6$

6) A swimming pool holds 2,000 cubic feet of water. The swimming pool is 25 feet long and 10 feet wide. How deep is the swimming pool?
   A. 2 *feet*
   B. 4 *feet*
   C. 6 *feet*
   D. 7 *feet*
   E. 8 *feet*

7) Mr. Carlos family are choosing a menu for their reception. They have 3 choices of appetizers, 7 choices of entrees, 4 choices of cake. How many different menu combinations are possible for them to choose?
   A. 12
   B. 32
   C. 84
   D. 120
   E. 240

8) What is the area of a square whose diagonal is 8?
   A. 16
   B. 32
   C. 36
   D. 64
   E. 124

9) The perimeter of a rectangular yard is 60 meters. What is its length if its width is twice its length?
   A. 10 *meters*
   B. 18 *meters*
   C. 20 *meters*
   D. 24 *meters*
   E. 36 *meters*

10) The average of 6 numbers is 12. The average of 4 of those numbers is 10. What is the average of the other two numbers?
    A. 10
    B. 12
    C. 14
    D. 16
    E. 24

11) The average of five numbers is 24. If a sixth number 42 is added, then, what is the new average?
    A. 25
    B. 26
    C. 27
    D. 28
    E. 36

12) The ratio of boys and girls in a class is $4:7$. If there are 66 students in the class, how many more boys should be enrolled to make the ratio $1:1$?

A. 8
B. 10
C. 12
D. 18
E. 28

13) Jason needs an 76% average in his writing class to pass. On his first 4 exams, he earned scores of 68%, 72%, 85%, and 90%. What is the minimum score Jason can earn on his fifth and final test to pass?

A. 80%,
B. 70%
C. 68%
D. 65%
E. 60%

14) 5 less than twice a positive integer is 53. What is the integer?

A. 29
B. 41
C. 42
D. 44
E. 53

15) A bank is offering 3.5% simple interest on a savings account. If you deposit $12,000, how much interest will you earn in two years?

A. $420
B. $840
C. $4,200
D. $8,400
E. $9,600

16) Simplify $6x^2y^3(2x^2y)^3 =$

A. $12x^4y^6$
B. $12x^8y^6$
C. $48x^4y^6$
D. $48x^8y^6$
E. $96x^8y^6$

17) The radius of the following cylinder is 6 inches and its height is 12 inches. What is the surface area of the cylinder in square inches?

    A. 567.98
    B. 640
    C. 678.24
    D. 888.25
    E. 910.21

18) A cruise line ship left Port A and traveled 80 miles due west and then 150 miles due north. At this point, what is the shortest distance from the cruise to port A?
    A. 70 $miles$
    B. 80 $miles$
    C. 150 $miles$
    D. 230 $miles$
    E. 170 $miles$

19) What is the equivalent temperature of 140°$F$ in Celsius?
$$C = \frac{5}{9}(F - 32)$$

    A. 32
    B. 40
    C. 48
    D. 52
    E. 60

20) If 150% of a number is 75, then what is the 95% of that number?
    A. 47.5
    B. 50
    C. 70
    D. 85
    E. 90

21) In two successive years, the population of a town is increased by 15% and 20%. What percent of the population is increased after two years?
    A. 32%
    B. 35%
    C. 38%
    D. 68%
    E. 70%

22) Last week 24,000 fans attended a football match. This week three times as many bought tickets, but one sixth of them cancelled their tickets. How many are attending this week?
   A. 48,000
   B. 54,000
   C. 60,000
   D. 72,000
   E. 84,000

23) What is the perimeter of a square that has an area of 64 square inches?
   A. 144 *inches*
   B. 64 *inches*
   C. 56 *inches*
   D. 48 *inches*
   E. 32 *inches*

24) In the $xy$-plane, the point $(4,3)$ and $(3,2)$ are on line A. Which of the following points could also be on line A?
   A. $(-1,2)$
   B. $(5,7)$
   C. $(3,4)$
   D. $(-1,-2)$
   E. $(-7,-9)$

25) If $f(x) = 2x^3 + 5x^2 + 2x$ and $g(x) = -2$, what is the value of $f(g(x))$?
   A. 36
   B. 32
   C. 24
   D. 4
   E. 0

26) The area of a circle is $64\pi$. What is the diameter of the circle?
   A. 4
   B. 8
   C. 12
   D. 14
   E. 16

27) If a tree casts a 22–foot shadow at the same time that a 3 feet yardstick casts a 2–foot shadow, what is the height of the tree?

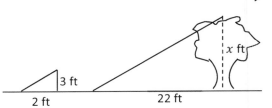

A. 24 $ft$
B. 28 $ft$
C. 33 $ft$
D. 98 $ft$
E. 108 $ft$

28) Which of the following is equal to the expression below?

$$(4x + 2y)(2x - y)$$

A. $8x^2 - 2y^2$
B. $2x^2 + 6xy - 2y^2$
C. $24x^2 + 2xy - 2y^2$
D. $8x^2 + 2xy - 2y^2$
E. $8x^2 + 2xy - 2y^2$

29) What is the product of all possible values of $x$ in the following equation?

$$|x - 10| = 3$$

A. 3
B. 7
C. 13
D. 91
E. 100

30) What is the slope of a line that is perpendicular to the line
$$4x - 2y = 12?$$

A. $-2$
B. $-\frac{1}{2}$
C. 4
D. 12
E. 14

31) What is the value of the expression $5(x - 2y) + (2 - x)^2$ when $x = 3$ and $= -2$ ?
A. $-4$
B. 20
C. 36
D. 50
E. 80

32) Jason is 15 miles ahead of Joe running at 5.5 miles per hour and Joe is running at the speed of 7 miles per hour. How long does it take Joe to catch Jason?
   A. 3 *hours*
   B. 4 *hours*
   C. 6 *hours*
   D. 8 *hours*
   E. 10 *hours*

33) 88 students took an exam and 11 of them failed. What percent of the students passed the exam?
   A. 20%
   B. 40.3%
   C. 60%
   D. 87.5%
   E. 90.15

34) If $tan\ \theta = \frac{5}{12}$ and $sin\ \theta > 0$, then $cos\ \theta = ?$
   A. $-\frac{5}{13}$
   B. $\frac{12}{13}$
   C. $\frac{13}{12}$
   D. $-\frac{12}{13}$
   E. 0

35) If the area of trapezoid is 100, what is the perimeter of the trapezoid?

   A. 25
   B. 35
   C. 45
   D. 55
   E. 65

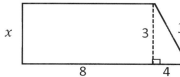

36) A number is chosen at random from 1 to 25. Find the probability of not selecting a composite number.

    A. $\dfrac{1}{25}$

    B. 25

    C. $\dfrac{2}{5}$

    D. 1

    E. 0

37) Removing which of the following numbers will change the average of the numbers to 6?

    1, 4, 5, 8, 11, 12

    A. 1

    B. 4

    C. 5

    D. 11

    E. 12

38) If $(x - 2)^2 + 1 > 3x - 1$, then $x$ can equal which of the following?

    A. 1

    B. 6

    C. 8

    D. 3

    E. 4

39) If 150% of a number is 75, then what is 90% of that number?

    A. 45

    B. 50

    C. 70

    D. 85

    E. 90

40) If one angle of a right triangle measures 60°, what is the sine of the other acute angle?

   A. $\frac{1}{2}$

   B. $\frac{\sqrt{2}}{2}$

   C. $\frac{\sqrt{3}}{2}$

   D. 1

   E. $\sqrt{3}$

## End of DAT Quantitative Reasoning Practice Test 4

# DAT Quantitative Reasoning Practice Test 5

## 2019 - 2020

**Total number of questions:** 40

**Total time:** 45 Minutes

**A basic four function calculator is permitted for DAT Quantitative Reasoning Test.**

# DAT Quantitative Reasoning Practice Tests Answer Sheet

**Remove (or photocopy) this answer sheet and use it to complete the practice tests.**

### DAT Quantitative Reasoning Practice Test Answer Sheet

DAT Quantitative Reasoning Practice Test 5

| | | | |
|---|---|---|---|
| 1 (A)(B)(C)(D)(E) | 16 (A)(B)(C)(D)(E) | 31 (A)(B)(C)(D)(E) | |
| 2 (A)(B)(C)(D)(E) | 17 (A)(B)(C)(D)(E) | 32 (A)(B)(C)(D)(E) | |
| 3 (A)(B)(C)(D)(E) | 18 (A)(B)(C)(D)(E) | 33 (A)(B)(C)(D)(E) | |
| 4 (A)(B)(C)(D)(E) | 19 (A)(B)(C)(D)(E) | 34 (A)(B)(C)(D)(E) | |
| 5 (A)(B)(C)(D)(E) | 20 (A)(B)(C)(D)(E) | 35 (A)(B)(C)(D)(E) | |
| 6 (A)(B)(C)(D)(E) | 21 (A)(B)(C)(D)(E) | 36 (A)(B)(C)(D)(E) | |
| 7 (A)(B)(C)(D)(E) | 22 (A)(B)(C)(D)(E) | 37 (A)(B)(C)(D)(E) | |
| 8 (A)(B)(C)(D)(E) | 23 (A)(B)(C)(D)(E) | 38 (A)(B)(C)(D)(E) | |
| 9 (A)(B)(C)(D)(E) | 24 (A)(B)(C)(D)(E) | 39 (A)(B)(C)(D)(E) | |
| 10 (A)(B)(C)(D)(E) | 25 (A)(B)(C)(D)(E) | 40 (A)(B)(C)(D)(E) | |
| 11 (A)(B)(C)(D)(E) | 26 (A)(B)(C)(D)(E) | | |
| 12 (A)(B)(C)(D)(E) | 27 (A)(B)(C)(D)(E) | | |
| 13 (A)(B)(C)(D)(E) | 28 (A)(B)(C)(D)(E) | | |
| 14 (A)(B)(C)(D)(E) | 29 (A)(B)(C)(D)(E) | | |
| 15 (A)(B)(C)(D)(E) | 30 (A)(B)(C)(D)(E) | | |

1) What is the value of the expression $2(2x - y) + (4 - x)^2$ when $x = 2$ and $y = -1$ ?
   A. $-2$
   B. $8$
   C. $14$
   D. $28$
   E. $50$

2) A swimming pool holds 1,500 cubic feet of water. The swimming pool is 15 feet long and 10 feet wide. How deep is the swimming pool?
   A. $2\ feet$
   B. $4\ feet$
   C. $6\ feet$
   D. $8\ feet$
   E. $10\ feet$

3) Mr. Carlos family are choosing a menu for their reception. They have 5 choices of appetizers, 4 choices of entrees, 3 choices of cake. How many different menu combinations are possible for them to choose?
   A. $12$
   B. $32$
   C. $60$
   D. $120$
   E. $240$

4) If $f(x) = x^3 - 2x^2 + 8x$ and $g(x) = 3$, what is the value of $f(g(x))$?
   A. $-3$
   B. $11$
   C. $22$
   D. $23$
   E. $33$

5) The diagonal of a rectangle is $10\ inches$ long and the height of the rectangle is $8\ inches$. What is the perimeter of the rectangle?
   A. $10\ inches$
   B. $12\ inches$
   C. $16\ inches$
   D. $18\ inches$
   E. $28\ inches$

6) The perimeter of the trapezoid below is $42\ cm$. What is its area?

  A.  $38\ cm^2$
  B.  $52.5\ cm^2$
  C.  $120\ cm^2$
  D.  $360\ cm^2$
  E.  $720\ cm^2$

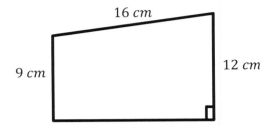

7) The average of seven numbers is 32. If an eighth number 18 is added, then, what is the new average?

  A.  24
  B.  28
  C.  30.25
  D.  32
  E.  34

8) The ratio of boys and girls in a class is $4:7$. If there are 44 students in the class, how many more boys should be enrolled to make the ratio $1:1$?

  A.  8
  B.  10
  C.  12
  D.  14
  E.  28

9) What is the value of $x$ in the following equation?

$$\frac{2}{3}x + \frac{1}{6} = \frac{1}{3}$$

  A.  $6$
  B.  $\frac{1}{2}$
  C.  $\frac{1}{3}$
  D.  $\frac{1}{4}$
  E.  $\frac{1}{12}$

10) A bank is offering 2.5% simple interest on a savings account. If you deposit $16,000, how much interest will you earn in three years?
   A. $610
   B. $1,200
   C. $2,400
   D. $4,800
   E. $6,400

11) Jason needs an 75% average in his writing class to pass. On his first 4 exams, he earned scores of 68%, 72%, 85%, and 90%. What is the minimum score Jason can earn on his fifth and final test to pass?
   A. 80%
   B. 70%
   C. 68%
   D. 64%
   E. 60%

12) Two dice are thrown simultaneously, what is the probability of getting a sum of 6 or 9?
   A. $\dfrac{1}{3}$
   B. $\dfrac{1}{12}$
   C. $\dfrac{1}{6}$
   D. $\dfrac{1}{4}$
   E. $\dfrac{1}{36}$

13) What is the surface area of the cylinder below?
   A. $48\pi\ in^2$
   B. $57\pi\ in^2$
   C. $66\pi\ in^2$
   D. $288\pi\ in^2$
   E. $400\pi\ in^2$

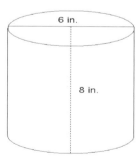

6 in.

8 in.

14) Which of the following is equal to the expression below?
$$(3x - y)(2x + 2y)$$
   A. $6x^2 - 2y^2$
   B. $6x^2 + 4xy + 2y^2$
   C. $12x^2 + 6xy + 2y^2$
   D. $6x^2 + 4xy - 2y^2$
   E. $4x^2 + 6xy - 2y^2$

15) What is the product of all possible values of $x$ in the following equation?

$$|x - 12| = 4$$

  A.  4
  B.  8
  C.  16
  D.  128
  E.  200

16) What is the slope of a line that is perpendicular to the line
$$4x - 2y = 12?$$

  A.  $-2$
  B.  $-\frac{1}{2}$
  C.  4
  D.  12
  E.  14

17) Last week 18,000 fans attended a football match. This week three times as many bought tickets, but one sixth of them cancelled their tickets. How many are attending this week?
  A.  42,000
  B.  54,000
  C.  45,000
  D.  65,000
  E.  78,000

18) What is the perimeter of a square that has an area of 81 square inches?
  A.  $129 \ inches$
  B.  $72 \ inches$
  C.  $68 \ inches$
  D.  $58 \ inches$
  E.  $36 \ inches$

19) What are the zeros of the function: $f(x) = x^2 - 7x + 12$?
  A.  0
  B.  $-2, -3$
  C.  $0, 4, 3$
  D.  $-4, -3$
  E.  $4, 3$

20) The mean of 50 test scores was calculated as 88. But, it turned out that one of the scores was misread as 94 but it was 69. What is the mean?
   A. 85
   B. 87
   C. 87.5
   D. 88.5
   E. 90.5

21) What is the equivalent temperature of $122°F$ in Celsius?
   $$C = \frac{5}{9}(F - 32)$$
   A. 22
   B. 50
   C. 58
   D. 62
   E. 84

22) The perimeter of a rectangular *yard* is 120 *meters*. What is its length if its width is twice its length?
   A. 20 *meters*
   B. 22 *meters*
   C. 24 *meters*
   D. 28 *meters*
   E. 30 *meters*

23) If 150% of a number is 75, then what is the 90% of that number?
   A. 45
   B. 50
   C. 70
   D. 85
   E. 90

24) What is the slope of the line: $8x - 4y = 8$

   A. $-1$
   B. $-2$
   C. 1
   D. 1.5
   E. 2

25) In two successive years, the population of a town is increased by 12% and 25%. What percent of the population is increased after two years?

    A.  34%
    B.  38%
    C.  40%
    D.  60%
    E.  80%

26) The average of 8 numbers is 14. The average of 6 of those numbers is 12. What is the average of the other two numbers?

    A.  12
    B.  14
    C.  16
    D.  20
    E.  28

27) Five years ago, Amy was three times as old as Mike was. If Mike is 10 years old now, how old is Amy?

    A.  4
    B.  8
    C.  12
    D.  14
    E.  20

28) If a tree casts a 18–foot shadow at the same time that a 4 feet yardstick casts a 3–foot shadow, what is the height of the tree?

    A.  18 $ft$
    B.  20 $ft$
    C.  24 $ft$
    D.  54 $ft$
    E.  62 $ft$

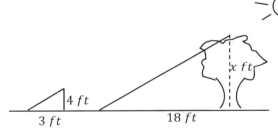

29) $x$ is $y$% of what number?

    A.  $\dfrac{100x}{y}$

    B.  $\dfrac{100y}{x}$

    C.  $\dfrac{x}{100y}$

    D.  $\dfrac{y}{100x}$

    E.  $\dfrac{xy}{100}$

30) If cotangent of an angel β is 1, then the tangent of angle β is

   A.  −1

   B.  0

   C.  1

   D.  2

   E.  3

31) 6 liters of water are poured into an aquarium that's 15cm long, 5cm wide, and 60cm high. How many cm will the water level in the aquarium rise due to this added water? (1 liter of water = 1000 cm3)

   A.  80

   B.  40

   C.  20

   D.  10

   E.  5

32) If a box contains red and blue balls in ratio of 2 : 3, how many red balls are there if 90 blue balls are in the box?

   A.  90

   B.  60

   C.  30

   D.  10

   E.  8

33) If $|a| < 1$, then which of the following is true? $(b > 0)$?

     I.  $-b < ba < b$

     II.  $-a < a^2 < a \quad if \ a < 0$

     III.  $-5 < 2a - 3 < -1$

   A.  I only

   B.  II only

   C.  I and III only

   D.  III only

   E.  I, II and III

34) A cruise line ship left Port $A$ and traveled 80 miles due west and then 150 miles due north. At this point, what is the shortest distance from the cruise to port $A$?
   A. 70 *miles*
   B. 80 *miles*
   C. 150 *miles*
   D. 230 *miles*
   E. 170 *miles*

35) If 30% of a number is 12, what is the number?
   A. 12
   B. 25
   C. 40
   D. 45
   E. 50

36) Jason is 15 miles ahead of Joe running at 4.5 miles per hour and Joe is running at the speed of 7 miles per hour. How long does it take Joe to catch Jason?
   A. 3 *hours*
   B. 4 *hours*
   C. 6 *hours*
   D. 8 *hours*
   E. 10 *hours*

37) 55 Students took an exam and 11 of them failed. What percent of the students passed the exam?
   A. 20%
   B. 40%
   C. 60%
   D. 80%
   E. 90%

38) The following table represents the value of $x$ and function $f(x)$. Which of the following could be the equation of the function $f(x)$?

   A. $f(x) = x^2 - 5$
   B. $f(x) = x^2 - 1$
   C. $f(x) = \sqrt{x+2}$
   D. $f(x) = \sqrt{x} + 4$
   D. $f(x) = \sqrt{x+1} + 4$

| $x$ | $f(x)$ |
|-----|--------|
| 1   | 5      |
| 4   | 6      |
| 9   | 7      |
| 16  | 8      |

39) In the following equation when $z$ is divided by 3, what is the effect on $x$?

$$x = \frac{8y + \dfrac{r}{r+1}}{\dfrac{6}{z}}$$

A. $x$ is divided by 2

B. $x$ is divided by 3

C. $x$ does not change

D. $x$ is multiplied by 3

E. $x$ is multiplied by 2

40) If $x \blacksquare y = \sqrt{x^2 + y}$, what is the value of $6 \blacksquare 28$?

A. $\sqrt{168}$
B. 10
C. 8
D. 6
E. 4.5

## End of DAT Quantitative Reasoning Practice Test 5

# DAT Quantitative Reasoning Practice Tests
## Answer Keys

Now, it's time to review your results to see where you went wrong and what areas you need to improve.

| DAT Quantitative Reasoning Practice Test 1 | | | | DAT Quantitative Reasoning Practice Test 2 | | | | DAT Quantitative Reasoning Practice Test 3 | | | |
|---|---|---|---|---|---|---|---|---|---|---|---|
| 1 | C | 21 | D | 1 | C | 21 | E | 1 | C | 21 | C |
| 2 | B | 22 | C | 2 | D | 22 | E | 2 | B | 22 | C |
| 3 | D | 23 | C | 3 | D | 23 | B | 3 | C | 23 | B |
| 4 | E | 24 | D | 4 | D | 24 | A | 4 | B | 24 | C |
| 5 | E | 25 | A | 5 | B | 25 | D | 5 | C | 25 | E |
| 6 | E | 26 | C | 6 | C | 26 | A | 6 | C | 26 | E |
| 7 | E | 27 | B | 7 | E | 27 | E | 7 | D | 27 | C |
| 8 | C | 28 | C | 8 | C | 28 | B | 8 | E | 28 | C |
| 9 | E | 29 | A | 9 | B | 29 | C | 9 | C | 29 | E |
| 10 | C | 30 | D | 10 | D | 30 | D | 10 | E | 30 | E |
| 11 | B | 31 | C | 11 | C | 31 | C | 11 | C | 31 | E |
| 12 | E | 32 | B | 12 | A | 32 | C | 12 | B | 32 | E |
| 13 | E | 33 | B | 13 | A | 33 | D | 13 | B | 33 | E |
| 14 | D | 34 | D | 14 | E | 34 | E | 14 | A | 34 | C |
| 15 | B | 35 | C | 15 | B | 35 | E | 15 | C | 35 | D |
| 16 | B | 36 | E | 16 | B | 36 | B | 16 | B | 36 | D |
| 17 | A | 37 | E | 17 | D | 37 | E | 17 | B | 37 | B |
| 18 | E | 38 | A | 18 | A | 38 | D | 18 | B | 38 | B |
| 19 | B | 39 | D | 19 | C | 39 | C | 19 | B | 39 | D |
| 20 | A | 40 | A | 20 | E | 40 | A | 20 | C | 40 | B |

| DAT Quantitative Reasoning Practice Test 4 | | | | DAT Quantitative Reasoning Practice Test 5 | | | |
|---|---|---|---|---|---|---|---|
| 1 | E | 21 | C | 1 | C | 21 | B |
| 2 | E | 22 | C | 2 | E | 22 | A |
| 3 | C | 23 | E | 3 | C | 23 | A |
| 4 | A | 24 | D | 4 | E | 24 | E |
| 5 | D | 25 | E | 5 | E | 25 | C |
| 6 | E | 26 | E | 6 | B | 26 | D |
| 7 | C | 27 | C | 7 | C | 27 | E |
| 8 | B | 28 | A | 8 | C | 28 | C |
| 9 | A | 29 | D | 9 | D | 29 | A |
| 10 | D | 30 | B | 10 | B | 30 | C |
| 11 | C | 31 | C | 11 | E | 31 | A |
| 12 | D | 32 | E | 12 | D | 32 | B |
| 13 | D | 33 | D | 13 | C | 33 | C |
| 14 | A | 34 | B | 14 | D | 34 | E |
| 15 | B | 35 | B | 15 | D | 35 | C |
| 16 | E | 36 | C | 16 | B | 36 | C |
| 17 | C | 37 | D | 17 | C | 37 | D |
| 18 | E | 38 | A | 18 | E | 38 | D |
| 19 | E | 39 | C | 19 | E | 39 | B |
| 20 | A | 40 | A | 20 | C | 40 | C |

# DAT Quantitative Reasoning Practice Tests

## Answers and Explanations

## DAT Quantitative Reasoning Practice Test 1

**1) Choice C is correct**

Add the first 5 numbers. $40 + 45 + 50 + 35 + 55 = 225$, To find the distance traveled in the next 5 hours, multiply the average by number of hours. $Distance = Average \times Rate = 65 \times 5 = 325$. Add both numbers. $325 + 225 = 550$

**2) Choice B is correct**

Use distance formula: $Distance = Rate \times time \Rightarrow 420 = 65 \times T$, divide both sides by $65$. $420 \div 65 = T \Rightarrow T = 6.4\ hours$. Change hours to minutes for the decimal part. $0.4\ hours = 0.4 \times 60 = 24\ minutes$.

**3) Choice D is correct**

Use Pythagorean Theorem: $a^2 + b^2 = c^2 \Rightarrow 5^2 + 12^2 = c^2 \Rightarrow 169 = c^2 \Rightarrow c = 13$

**4) Choice E is correct**

Th ratio of boy to girls is $2 : 3$. Therefore, there are 2 boys out of 5 students. To find the answer, first divide the total number of students by 5, then multiply the result by 2.

$500 \div 5 = 100 \Rightarrow 100 \times 2 = 200$

**5) Choice E is correct**

Use FOIL (First, Out, In, Last). $(7x + 2y)(5x + 2y) = 35x^2 + 14xy + 10xy + 4y^2 =$

$$35x^2 + 24xy + 4y^2$$

**6) Choice E is correct**

Use distributive property: $5x(4 + 2y) = 20x + 10xy$

**7) Choice E is correct**

$y = 5ab + 3b^3$. Plug in the values of $a$ and $b$ in the equation: $a = 2$ and $b = 3$.

$y = 5\,(2)(3) + 3\,(3)^3 = 30 + 3(27) = 30 + 81 = 111$

**8) Choice C is correct**

$x = \frac{15}{20} = 0.75 = 75\%$.

**9) Choice E is correct**

The perimeter of the trapezoid is 64. Therefore, the missing side (height) is

$= 64 - 18 - 12 - 14 = 20$. Area of the trapezoid: $A = \frac{1}{2} h (b_1 + b_2) =$

$$\frac{1}{2} (20) (12 + 14) = 260$$

**10) Choice C is correct**

Let $x$ be the number. Write the equation and solve for $x$. $\frac{2}{3} \times 15 = \frac{2}{5} . x \Rightarrow \frac{2 \times 15}{3} = \frac{2x}{5}$ , use cross multiplication to solve for $x$. $5 \times 30 = 2x \times 3 \Rightarrow 150 = 6x \Rightarrow x = 25$

**11) Choice B is correct**

To find the discount, multiply the number by $(100\% - rate\ of\ discount)$.

Therefore, for the first discount we get: $(D) (100\% - 25\%) = (D)(0.75) = 0.75\ D$

For increase of 10%: $(0.75\ D)(100\% + 10\%) = (0.75\ D)(1.10) = 0.82\ D = 82\%\ of\ D$

**12) Choice E is correct**

Surface Area of a cylinder $= 2\pi r\ (r + h)$, The radius of the cylinder is 8 inches and its height is 14 inches. Surface Area of a cylinder $= 2\ (\pi)(8)(8 + 14) = 352\ \pi$

**13) Choice E is correct**

$$\text{average} = \frac{\text{sum of terms}}{\text{number of terms}} \Rightarrow 20 = \frac{13 + 15 + 20 + x}{4} \Rightarrow 80 = 48 + x \Rightarrow x = 32$$

**14) Choice D is correct**

Let $x$ be the original price. If the price of the sofa is decreased by 25% to $450, then: $75\%\ of\ x = 450 \Rightarrow 0.75x = 450 \Rightarrow x = 450 \div 0.75 = 600$

**15) Choice B is correct**

Use the formula of areas of circles. $Area = \pi r^2 \Rightarrow 49\pi = \pi r^2 \Rightarrow 49 = r^2 \Rightarrow r = 7$

Radius of the circle is 7. Now, use the circumference formula: Circumference $=$

$2\pi r = 2\pi\ (7) = 14\ \pi$.

**16) Choice B is correct**

Use the formula for Percent of Change. $\frac{\text{New Value}-\text{Ol} \ \text{Value}}{\text{Old Value}} \times 100\%$ .

$\frac{28-50}{50} \times 100 \% = -44\%$ (negative sign here means that the new price is less than old price).

**17) Choice A is correct**

Let $x$ be the number of years. Therefore, $2,000 per year equals $2000x$. starting from $26,000 annual salary means you should add that amount to $2000x$. Income more than that is:

$I > 2000 \ x \ + \ 26000$

**18) Choice E is correct**

Use the information provided in the question to draw the shape.

Use Pythagorean Theorem: $a^2 + b^2 = c^2$

$60^2 + 80^2 = c^2 \Rightarrow 3600 + 6400 = c^2 \Rightarrow 10000 = c^2 \Rightarrow c = 100$

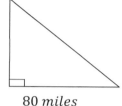

60 *miles*

80 *miles*

**19) Choice B is correct**

The question is this: 530.40 is what percent of 631?

$percent = \frac{530.40}{631} = 84.05 \cong 84$. 530.40 is 84% of 631. Therefore, the discount is:

$100\% - 84\% = 16\%$

**20) Choice A is correct**

If the score of Mia was 40, therefore the score of Ava is 20. Since, the score of Emma was half as that of Ava, therefore, the score of Emma is 10.

**21) Choice D is correct**

If 17 balls are removed from the bag at random, there will be one ball in the bag. The probability of choosing a brown ball is 1 out of 18. Therefore, the probability of not choosing a brown ball is 17 out of 18 and the probability of having not a brown ball after removing 17 balls is the same.

**22) Choice C is correct**

Let $x$ be the smallest number. Then, these are the numbers: $x, x + 1, x + 2, x + 3, x + 4$

$\text{average} = \frac{\text{sum of terms}}{\text{number of terms}} \Rightarrow 36 = \frac{x+(x+1)+(x+2)+(x+3)+(x+4)}{5} \Rightarrow 36 = \frac{5x+10}{5} \Rightarrow$

$180 = 5x + 10 \Rightarrow 170 = 5x \Rightarrow x = 34$

**23) Choice C is correct**

Use this formula: Percent of Change: $\frac{\text{New Value}-\text{Old Value}}{\text{Old Value}} \times 100\%$ .

$\dfrac{18,200-28,000}{28,000} \times 100\% = -35\%$. The negative sign means that the price decreased

### 24) Choice D is correct

If the length of the box is 36, then the width of the box is one third of it, 12, and the height of the box is 4 (one third of the width). The volume of the box is: $V = lwh = (36)(12)(4) = 1,728$

### 25) Choice A is correct

Write a proportion and solve for the missing number. $\dfrac{32}{12} = \dfrac{6}{x} \rightarrow 32x = 6 \times 12 = 72$

$$32x = 72 \rightarrow x = \dfrac{72}{32} = 2.25$$

### 26) Choice C is correct

Let $x$ be the number. Write the equation and solve for $x$. $(28 - x) \div x = 3$

Multiply both sides by $x$. $(28 - x) = 3x$, then add $x$ both sides. $28 = 4x$, now divide both sides by 4. $x = 7$

### 27) Choice B is correct

The sum of supplement angles is 180. Let $x$ be that angle. Therefore, $x + 9x = 180$

$10x = 180$, divide both sides by 10: $x = 18$

### 28) Choice C is correct

The average speed of john is: $150 \div 6 = 25$, The average speed of Alice is: $140 \div 4 = 35$

Write the ratio and simplify. $25 : 35 \Rightarrow 5 : 7$

### 29) Choice A is correct

The percent of girls playing tennis is: $45\% \times 25\% = 0.45 \times 0.25 = 0.11 = 11\%$

### 30) Choice D is correct

The area of the floor is: $7\ cm \times 24\ cm = 168\ cm^2$, The number is tiles needed $=$

$168 \div 8 = 21$.

### 31) Choice C is correct

The weight of 14.2 meters of this rope is: $14.2 \times 600\ g = 8520\ g$

$1\ kg = 1000\ g$, therefore, $8520\ g \div 1,000 = 8.52\ kg$

### 32) Choice B is correct

6% of the volume of the solution is alcohol. Let $x$ be the volume of the solution.

Then: $6\% \ of \ x = 24 \ ml \Rightarrow 0.06 \ x = 24 \Rightarrow x = 24 \div 0.06 = 400$

### 33) Choice B is correct

average $= \frac{\text{sum of terms}}{\text{number of terms}}$. The sum of the weight of all girls is: $18 \times 56 = 1,008 \ kg$

The sum of the weight of all boys is: $32 \times 62 = 1,984 \ kg$.The sum of the weight of all students is: $1,008 + 1,984 = 2,992 \ kg$. $average = \frac{2992}{50} = 59.84$

### 34) Choice D is correct

Let $x$ be the original price. If the price of a laptop is decreased by 20% to $360, then: $80\% \ of$

$x = 360 \Rightarrow 0.80x = 360 \Rightarrow x = 360 \div 0.80 = 450$

### 35) Choice C is correct

Use simple interest formula: $I = prt$. (I = interest, p = principal, r = rate, t = time). $I = (9,000)(0.045)(5) = 2,025$

### 36) Choice E is correct

$(2.9 \times 10^6) \times (2.6 \times 10^{-5}) = (2.9 \times 2.6) \times (10^6 \times 10^{-5}) = 7.54 \times (10^{6+(-5)})$
$$= 7.54 \times 10^1$$

### 37) Choice E is correct

The formula of the volume of pyramid is: $V = \frac{l \times w \times h}{3}$

The length and width of the pyramid is $6 \ cm$ and its height is $14 \ cm$. Therefore:

$$V = \frac{6 \times 6 \times 14}{3} = 168 \ cm^3$$

### 38) Choice A is correct

Let $x$ be the integer. Then: $2x - 5 = 73$, Add 5 both sides: $2x = 78$, Divide both sides by 2:

$$x = 39$$

### 39) Choice D is correct

To find the discount, multiply the number by $(100\% - ate \ of \ discount)$.Therefore, for the first discount we get: $(300)(100\% - 15\%) = (300)(0.85)$. For the next $15\%$ discount: $(300)(0.85)(0.85)$.

### 40) Choice A is correct

Plug in each pair of number in the equation: $2x + 4y = 8$

A. $(2, 1)$:     $2(2) + 4(1) = 8$
B. $(-1, 3)$:     $2(-1) + 4(3) = 10$
C. $(-2, 2)$:     $2(-2) + 4(2) = 4$
D. $(2, 2)$:     $2(2) + 4(2) = 12$
E. $(2, 8)$:     $2(2) + 4(8) = 36$

Only choice A is correct.

# DAT Quantitative Reasoning Practice Test 2

**1) Choice C is correct**

$$average \ (mean) = \frac{sum \ of \ terms}{number \ of \ terms} \Rightarrow 90 = \frac{sum \ of \ terms}{50} \Rightarrow sum = 90 \times 50 = 4500$$

The difference of 94 and 69 is 25. Therefore, 25 should be subtracted from the sum.

$$4500 - 25 = 4475, mean = \frac{sum \ of \ terms}{number \ of \ terms} \Rightarrow mean = \frac{4475}{50} = 89.5$$

**2) Choice D is correct**

For sum of 5: (1 & 4) $and$ (4 & 1), (2 & 3) and (3 & 2), therefore we have 4 options.
For sum of 8: (5 & 3)$and$ (3 & 5), (4 & 4) and (2 & 6), and (6 & 2),we have 5 options. To get a sum of 5 or 8 for two dice: $4 + 5 = 9$.Since, we have $6 \times 6 = 36$ total number of options, the probability of getting a sum of 5 and 8 is 9 out of 36 or $\frac{9}{36} = \frac{1}{4}$

**3) Choice D is correct**

Use FOIL method. $(5x + 2y)(2x - y) = 10x^2 - 5xy + 4xy - 2y^2 = 10x^2 - xy - 2y^2$

**4) Choice D is correct**

To solve absolute values equations, write two equations. $x - 10$ could be positive 4, or negative 4. Therefore, $x - 10 = 4 \Rightarrow x = 14$, $x - 10 = -4 \Rightarrow x = 6$. Find the product of solutions: $6 \times 14 = 84$

**5) Choice B is correct**

The equation of a line in slope intercept form is: $y = \mathrm{m}x + b$. Solve for $y$.

$4x - 2y = 6 \Rightarrow -2y = 6 - 4x \Rightarrow y = (6 - 4x) \div (-2) \Rightarrow y = 2x - 3$. The slope is 2.

The slope of the line perpendicular to this line is: $m_1 \times m_2 = -1 \Rightarrow 2 \times m_2 = -1 \Rightarrow m_2 = -\frac{1}{2}$.

**6) Choice C is correct**

Plug in the value of $x$ and $y$. $x = 3$ and $y = -2$.

$6(x - 2y) + (2 - x)^2 = 6(3 - 2(-2)) + (2 - 3)^2 = 6(3 + 4) + (-1)^2 = 42 + 1 = 43$

**7) Choice E is correct**

Use formula of rectangle prism volume.$V = (length) \ (width) \ (height) \Rightarrow 2500 = (25) \ (10) \ (height) \Rightarrow height = 2500 \div 250 = 10$

**8) Choice C is correct**

$$4 \div \frac{1}{3} = 12$$

**9) Choice B is correct**

The diagonal of the square is 4. Let $x$ be the side. Use Pythagorean Theorem: $a^2 + b^2 = c^2$

$x^2 + x^2 = 4^2 \Rightarrow 2x^2 = 4^2 \Rightarrow 2x^2 = 16 \Rightarrow x^2 = 8 \Rightarrow x = \sqrt{8}$

The area of the square is: $\sqrt{8} \times \sqrt{8} = 8$

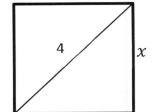

**10) Choice D is correct**

Solve for the sum of five numbers.

$$\text{average} = \frac{\text{sum of terms}}{\text{number of terms}} \Rightarrow 26 = \frac{sum\ of\ 5\ numbers}{5} \Rightarrow sum\ of\ 5\ numbers = 26 \times 5 = 130$$

The sum of 5 numbers is 130. If a sixth number 42 is added, then the sum of 6 numbers is

$130 + 42 = 172.\ average = \frac{\text{sum of terms}}{\text{number of terms}} = \frac{172}{6} = 28.66$

**11) Choice C is correct**

Th ratio of boy to girls is $4 : 7$. Therefore, there are 4 boys out of 11 students. To find the answer, first divide the total number of students by 11, then multiply the result by 4.

$55 \div 11 = 5 \Rightarrow 5 \times 4 = 20$. There are 20 boys and 35 $(55 - 20)$ girls. So, 15 more boys should be enrolled to make the ratio $1 : 1$

**12) Choice A is correct**

2,500 out of 65,000 equals to $\frac{2500}{65000} = \frac{25}{650} = \frac{1}{26}$

**13) Choice A is correct**

Let $x$ be the number of shoes the team can purchase. Therefore, the team can purchase $110\,x$.

The team had \$20,000 and spent \$14000. Now the team can spend on new shoes \$6000 at most. Now, write the inequality: $110x + 14,000 \le 20,000$

**14) Choice E is correct**

Jason needs an 70% average to pass for five exams. Therefore, the sum of 5 exams must be at lease $5 \times 70 = 350$. The sum of 4 exams is: $68 + 72 + 85 + 90 = 315$.

The minimum score Jason can earn on his fifth and final test to pass is: $350 - 315 = 35$

**15) Choice B is correct**

Isolate and solve for $x . \frac{2}{3}x + \frac{1}{6} = \frac{1}{2} \Rightarrow \frac{2}{3}x = \frac{1}{2} - \frac{1}{6} = \frac{1}{3} \Rightarrow \frac{2}{3}x = \frac{1}{3}$ .Multiply both sides by the reciprocal of the coefficient of $x$. $(\frac{3}{2}) \frac{1}{3} x = \frac{1}{3} (\frac{3}{2}) \Rightarrow x = \frac{3}{6} = \frac{1}{2}$

**16) Choice B is correct**

Use simple interest formula: $I = prt$ ($I$ = interest, $p$ = principal, $r$ = rate, $t$ = time).

$$I = (12,000)(0.045)(2) = 1,080$$

**17) Choice D is correct**

Simplify. $7x^2 y^3 (2x^2 y)^3 = 7x^2 y^3 (8x^6 y^3) = 56x^8 y^6$

**18) Choice A is correct**

Surface Area of a cylinder $= 2\pi r (r + h)$, The radius of the cylinder is 2 ($4 \div 2$) inches and its height is 8 inches. Therefore, Surface Area of a cylinder $= 2\pi (2) (2 + 8) = 40\pi$

**19) Choice C is correct**

Three times of 25,000 is 75,000. One sixth of them cancelled their tickets. One sixth of 75,000 equals 12,500 ($\frac{1}{6} \times 75000 = 12500$). 62,500 ($75000 - 12000 = 62500$) fans are attending this week.

**20) Choice E is correct**

The area of the square is 49 inches. Therefore, the side of the square is square root of the area.

$\sqrt{49} = 7$ inches. Four times the side of the square is the perimeter: $4 \times 7 = 28 \, inches$

**21) Choice E is correct**

$g(x) = -4$, then $f(g(x)) = f(-4) = 2(-4)^3 + 5(-4)^2 + 2(-4) = -128 + 80 - 8 = -56$

**22) Choice E is correct**

Use the information provided in the question to draw the shape.

Use Pythagorean Theorem: $a^2 + b^2 = c^2$

$50^2 + 120^2 = c^2 \Rightarrow 2,500 + 14,400 = c^2 \Rightarrow 16,900 = c^2 \Rightarrow c = 130$

**23) Choice B is correct**

Plug in 104 for $F$ and then solve for $C$.

$$C = \frac{5}{9} (F - 32) \Rightarrow C = \frac{5}{9} (104 - 32) \Rightarrow C = \frac{5}{9} (72) = 40$$

120 *miles*

Port A

50 *miles*

**24) Choice A is correct**

The width of the rectangle is twice its length. Let $x$ be the length. Then, $width = 2x$

Perimeter of the rectangle is $2\ (width\ +\ length) =\ 2(2x + x) = 72 \Rightarrow 6x = 72 \Rightarrow x = 12$. Length of the rectangle is 12 meters.

### 25) Choice D is correct

$average\ =\ \frac{sum\ of\ terms}{number\ of\ terms} \Rightarrow$ (average of 6 numbers) $14 = \frac{sum\ of\ numbers}{6} \Rightarrow$ sum of 6 numbers is $14 \times 6 = 84$, (average of 4 numbers) $10 = \frac{sum\ of\ numbers}{4} \Rightarrow$ sum of 4 numbers is $10 \times 4 = 40$. $sum\ of\ 6\ numbers\ -\ sum\ of\ 4\ numbers\ =\ sum\ of\ 2\ numbers$,

$84 - 40 = 44$ average of 2 numbers $= \frac{44}{2} = 22$

### 26) Choice A is correct

First, find the number. Let $x$ be the number. Write the equation and solve for $x$. 150% of a number is 75, then:$1.5 \times x = 75 \Rightarrow x = 75 \div 1.5 = 50, 80\%$ of 50 is:$0.8 \times 50 = 40$

### 27) Choice E is correct

Solve for $y$.$4x - 2y = 12 \Rightarrow -2y = 12 - 4x \Rightarrow y = 2x - 6$. The slope of the line is 2.

### 28) Choice B is correct

the population is increased by 10% and 20%. 10% increase changes the population to 110% of original population. For the second increase, multiply the result by 120%.

$(1.10) \times (1.20) = 1.32 = 132\%$. 32 percent of the population is increased after two years.

### 29) Choice C is correct

The formula for the area of the circle is: $A = \pi r^2$ ,The area is $36\pi$. Therefore:$A = \pi r^2 \Rightarrow 6\pi = \pi r^2$, Divide both sides by $\pi$: $36 = r^2 \Rightarrow r = 6$. Diameter of a circle is $2 \times$ radius. Then:

$Diameter = 2 \times 6 = 12$

### 30) Choice D is correct

If 20% of a number is 4, what is the number: $20\%\ of\ x = 4 \Rightarrow 0.20\ x = 4 \Rightarrow x = 4 \div 0.20 = 20$

### 31) Choice C is correct

Write a proportion and solve for $x$.$\frac{3}{2} = \frac{x}{26} \Rightarrow 2x = 3 \times 26 \Rightarrow x = 39\ ft$

### 32) Choice C is correct

The distance between Jason and Joe is $9\ miles$. Jason running at $6.5\ miles\ per\ hour$ and Joe is running at the speed of $8\ miles\ per\ hour$. Therefore, every hour the distance is $1.5\ miles$ less.

$9 \div 1.5 = 6$

**33) Choice D is correct**

The failing rate is 11 out of $44 = \frac{11}{44}$,Change the fraction to percent:$\frac{11}{44} \times 100\% = 25\%$. 25 percent of students failed. Therefore, 75 percent of students passed the exam.

**34) Choice E is correct**

$g(x) = -3$, then $f\big(g(x)\big) = f(-3) = 2\,(-3)^3 + 5(-3)^2 + 2(-3) = -54 + 45 - 6 = -15$

**35) Choice E is correct**

Let $x$ be the width of the rectangle. Use Pythagorean Theorem:

$a^2 + b^2 = c^2$

$x^2 + 6^2 = 10^2 \Rightarrow x^2 + 36 = 100 \Rightarrow x^2 = 100 - 36 = 64 \Rightarrow x = 8$

Perimeter of the rectangle $= 2\,(length + width) = 2\,(8 + 6) = 2\,(14) = 28$

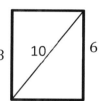

**36) Choice B is correct**

The perimeter of the trapezoid is 40.herefore, the missing side (height) is

$= 40 - 8 - 12 - 6 = 14$. Area of a trapezoid: $A = \frac{1}{2}\,h\,(b_1 + b_2) = \frac{1}{2}\,(14)\,(6 + 8) = 98$

**37) Choice E is correct**

$f\big(g(x)\big) = 2 \times (\frac{1}{x})^3 + 2 = \frac{2}{x^3} + 2$

**38) Choice D is correct**

Use the information provided in the question to draw the shape.

Use Pythagorean Theorem: $a^2 + b^2 = c^2$

$80^2 + 150^2 = c^2 \Rightarrow 6400 + 22500 = c^2 \Rightarrow 28900 = c^2 \Rightarrow c = 170$

1500 miles

Port A

80 miles

**39) Choice C is correct**

Write the ratio of $5a$ to $2b$. $\frac{5a}{2b} = \frac{1}{10}$. Use cross multiplication and then simplify.

$$5a \times 10 = 2b \times 1 \rightarrow 50a = 2b \rightarrow a = \frac{2b}{50} = \frac{b}{25}$$

Now, find the ratio of $a$ to $b$. $\frac{a}{b} = \frac{\frac{b}{25}}{b} \rightarrow \frac{b}{25} \div b = \frac{b}{25} \times \frac{1}{b} = \frac{b}{25} = \frac{1}{25}$

**40) Choice A is correct**

Plug in the value of $x$ in the equation and solve for $y$. $2y = \frac{2x^2}{3} + 6 \rightarrow 2y = \frac{2(9)^2}{3} + 6 \rightarrow$

$$2y = \frac{2(81)}{3} + 6 \rightarrow 2y = 54 + 6 = 60 \rightarrow 2y = 60 \rightarrow y = 30$$

# DAT Quantitative Reasoning Practice Test 3

### 1) Choice C is correct

Let $x$ be the number. Write the equation and solve for $x$. $(24 - x) \div x = 3$. Multiply both sides by $x$. $(24 - x) = 3x$, then add x both sides. $24 = 4x$, now divide both sides by 4.

$x = 6$

### 2) Choice B is correct

The sum of supplement angles is 180. Let $x$ be that angle. Therefore, $x + 5x = 180$

$6x = 180$, divide both sides by 6: $x = 30$

### 3) Choice C is correct

The average speed of john is: $150 \div 6 = 25$, The average speed of Alice is: $180 \div 4 = 45$

Write the ratio and simplify. $25 : 45 \Rightarrow 5 : 9$

### 4) Choice B is correct

The percent of girls playing tennis is: $40\% \times 35\% = 0.40 \times 0.35 = 0.14 = 14\%$

### 5) Choice C is correct

Add the first 5 numbers. $40 + 45 + 50 + 35 + 55 = 225$

To find the distance traveled in the next 5 hours, multiply the average by number of hours.

$Distance = Average \times Rate = 50 \times 5 = 250$, Add both numbers. $250 + 225 = 475$

### 6) Choice C is correct

Use distance formula: $Distance = Rate \times time \Rightarrow 420 = 50 \times T$, divide both sides by 50. $420 \div 50 = T \Rightarrow T = 8.4 \ hours$. Change hours to minutes for the decimal part. $0.4 \ hours = 0.4 \times 60 = 24 \ minutes$.

### 7) Choice D is correct

Use Pythagorean Theorem: $a^2 + b^2 = c^2$, $6^2 + 8^2 = c^2 \Rightarrow 100 = c^2 \Rightarrow c = 10$

### 8) Choice E is correct

Th ratio of boy to girls is $2 : 3$. Therefore, there are 2 boys out of 5 students. To find the answer, first divide the total number of students by 5, then multiply the result by 2.

$600 \div 5 = 120 \Rightarrow 120 \times 2 = 240$

### 9) Choice C is correct

Use percent formula: $part = \frac{percent}{100} \times whole$

$$25 = \frac{percent}{100} \times 20 \Rightarrow 25 = \frac{percent \times 20}{100} \Rightarrow 25$$
$$= \frac{percent \times 2}{10}, multiply\ both\ sides\ by\ 10.$$

$250 = percent \times 2$, divide both sides by 2. $125 = percent$

**10) Choice E is correct**

The perimeter of the trapezoid is 54.

Therefore, the missing side (height) is = $54 - 18 - 12 - 14 = 10$

Area of the trapezoid: $A = \frac{1}{2} h (b_1 + b_2) = \frac{1}{2} (10) (12 + 14) = 130$

**11) Choice C is correct**

Let $x$ be the number. Write the equation and solve for $x$.

$\frac{2}{3} \times 18 = \frac{2}{5} \cdot x \Rightarrow \frac{2 \times 18}{3} = \frac{2x}{5}$ , use cross multiplication to solve for $x$.

$5 \times 36 = 2x \times 3 \Rightarrow 180 = 6x \Rightarrow x = 30$

**12) Choice B is correct**

To find the discount, multiply the number by $(100\% - rate\ of\ discount)$.

Therefore, for the first discount we get: $(D) (100\% - 20\%) = (D) (0.80) = 0.80\ D$

For increase of 10%: $(0.80\ D)(100\% + 10\%) = (0.80\ D)(1.10) = 0.88\ D = 88\%\ of\ D$

**13) Choice B is correct**

Use the formula of areas of circles. $Area = \pi r^2 \Rightarrow 25\ \pi = \pi r^2 \Rightarrow 25 = r^2 \Rightarrow r = 5$

Radius of the circle is 5. Now, use the circumference formula: Circumference $= 2\pi r = 2\pi (5) = 10\ \pi$

**14) Choice A is correct**

Let $x$ be the number of years. Therefore, $3,000 per year equals $2000x$. starting from $24,000 annual salary means you should add that amount to $3000x$. Income more than that is:

$I > 3000\ x + 24000$

**15) Choice C is correct**

The question is this: 1.75 is what percent of 1.25? Use percent formula:

$$\text{part} = \frac{\text{percent}}{100} \times \text{whole}$$

$$1.75 = \frac{percent}{100} \times 1.25 \Rightarrow 1.75 = \frac{percent \times 1.25}{100} \Rightarrow 175 = percent \times 1.25$$

$$\Rightarrow percent = \frac{175}{1.25} = 140$$

### 16) Choice B is correct

Use the information provided in the question to draw the shape.

Use Pythagorean Theorem: $a^2 + b^2 = c^2$

$$40^2 + 30^2 = c^2 \Rightarrow 1600 + 900 = c^2 \Rightarrow 2500 = c^2 \Rightarrow c = 50$$

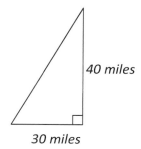

*40 miles*

*30 miles*

### 17) Choice B is correct

The question is this: 530.40 is what percent of 624?

Use percent formula: $\text{part} = \frac{\text{percent}}{100} \times \text{whole}$

$$530.40 = \frac{percent}{100} \times 624 \Rightarrow 530.40 = \frac{percent \times 624}{100} \Rightarrow 53040 = percent \times 624 \Rightarrow$$

$$percent = \frac{53040}{624} = 85$$

530.40 is 85% of 624. Therefore, the discount is: $100\% - 85\% = 15\%$

### 18) Choice B is correct

If the score of Mia was 60, therefore the score of Ava is 30. Since, the score of Emma was half as that of Ava, therefore, the score of Emma is 15.

### 19) Choice B is correct

Let $x$ be the smallest number. Then, these are the numbers: $x, x + 1, x + 2, x + 3, x + 4$

$average = \frac{\text{sum of terms}}{\text{number of terms}} \Rightarrow 38 = \frac{x+(x+1)+(x+2)+(x+3)+(x+4)}{5} \Rightarrow 38 = \frac{5x+10}{5} \Rightarrow 190 = 5x + 10 \Rightarrow 180 = 5x \Rightarrow x = 36$

### 20) Choice C is correct

The area of the floor is: $6 \, cm \times 24 \, cm = 144 \, cm^2$, The number is tiles needed $= 144 \div 8 = 18$

### 21) Choice C is correct

The weight of 12.2 meters of this rope is: $12.2 \times 600 \, g = 7320 \, g$,

$1 \, kg = 1000 \, g$, therefore, $7320 \, g \div 1000 = 7.32 \, kg$

**22) Choice C is correct**

4% of the volume of the solution is alcohol. Let $x$ be the volume of the solution.

Then: $4\% \ of \ x = 24 \ ml \Rightarrow 0.04 \ x = 24 \Rightarrow x = 24 \div 0.04 = 600$

**23) Choice B is correct**

$average = \frac{sum \ of \ terms}{number \ of \ terms}$, The sum of the weight of all girls is: $18 \times 60 = 1080 \ kg$, The sum of the weight of all boys is: $32 \times \ 62 = 1984 \ kg$, The sum of the weight of all students is: $1080 \ + \ 1984 \ = 3064 \ kg$, average $= \frac{3064}{50} = 61.28$

**24) Choice C is correct**

Let $x$ be the original price. If the price of a laptop is decreased by 10% to \$360, then: $90\% \ of \ x = 360 \Rightarrow 0.90x = 360 \Rightarrow x = 360 \div 0.90 = 400$

**25) Choice E is correct**

Surface Area of a cylinder $= 2\pi r \ (r + \ h)$, The radius of the cylinder is 8 inches and its height is 12 inches. Surface Area of a cylinder = $2 \ (\pi) \ (8) \ (8 + 12) = 320 \ \pi$

**26) Choice E is correct**

$average = \frac{sum \ of \ terms}{number \ of \ terms} \Rightarrow 18 = \frac{13+15+20+x}{4} \Rightarrow 72 \ = \ 48 \ + \ x \Rightarrow x = \ 24$

**27) Choice C is correct**

Let $x$ be the original price. If the price of the sofa is decreased by 25% to \$420, then: $75\% \ of \ x = 420 \Rightarrow 0.75x = 420 \Rightarrow x = 420 \div 0.75 = 560$

**28) Choice C is correct**

Use simple interest formula: $I = prt$, ($I$ = interest, $p$ = principal, $r \ $ = rate, $t \ $ = time)

$I = (8,000)(0.045)(5) = 1,800$

**29) Choice E is correct**

$$(4.2 \ \times \ 10^6) \ \times \ (2.6 \ \times \ 10^{-5}) = (4.2 \ \times \ 2.6) \times (10^6 \ \times \ 10^{-5}) = 10.92 \ \times \ (10^{6 \ + \ (-5)} \ )$$
$$= \ 1.092 \ \times \ 10^2$$

**30) Choice E is correct**

The formula of the volume of pyramid is: $V = \frac{l \ \times w \ \times h}{3}$. The length and width of the pyramid is $6 \ cm$ and its height is $12 \ cm$. Therefore: $V = \frac{6 \times 6 \ \times 12}{3} = 144 \ cm^3$

**31) Choice E is correct**

Simplify: $4(x + 1) = 6(x - 4) + 20, 4x + 4 = 6x - 24 + 20, 4x + 4 = 6x - 4$

Subtract $4x$ from both sides: $4 = 2x - 4$, Add 4 to both sides: $8 = 2x, 4 = x$

**32) Choice E is correct**

Use distributive property: $2x(4 + 2y) = 8x + 4xy = 4xy + 8x$

**33) Choice E is correct**

$y = 4ab + 3b^3$, plug in the values of $a$ and $b$ in the equation: $a = 2$ and $b = 3$,

$y = 4(2)(3) + 3(3)^3 = 24 + 3(27) = 24 + 81 = 105$

**34) Choice C is correct**

$11 \times 36 + 6 \times 12 + 4 = 472$

**35) Choice D is correct**

Let $x$ be the integer. Then: $2x - 5 = 83$, Add 5 both sides: $2x = 88$, Divide both sides by 2: $x = 44$

**36) Choice D is correct**

To find the discount, multiply the number by $(100\% - rate\ of\ discount)$. Therefore, for the first discount we get: $(200)(100\% - 15\%) = (200)(0.85)$, For the next 15% discount: $(200)(0.85)(0.85)$ .

**37) Choice B is correct**

Plug in each pair of number in the equation:

A. $(2, 1)$:      $2(2) + 4(1) = 8$
B. $(-1, 3)$:    $2(-1) + 4(3) = 10$
C. $(-2, 2)$:    $2(-2) + 4(2) = 4$
D. $(2, 2)$:      $2(2) + 4(2) = 12$

**38) Choice B is correct**

Use this formula: Percent of Change: $\dfrac{New\ Value - Old\ Value}{Old\ Value} \times 100\%$

$\dfrac{16000 - 20000}{20000} \times 100\% = -20\%$ and $\dfrac{12800 - 16000}{16000} \times 100\% = -20\%$

**39) Choice D is correct**

The relationship among all sides of special right triangle

$30° - 60° - 90°$ is provided in this triangle:

In this triangle, the opposite side of $30°$ angle is half of the hypotenuse.

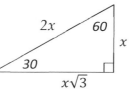
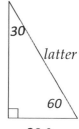

Draw the shape of this question:

The latter is the hypotenuse. Therefore, the latter is $60 \, ft$

**40) Choice B is correct.**

By definition, the sine of any acute angle is equal to the cosine of its complement.

Since, angle A and B are complementary angles, therefore: $\sin A = \cos B$

# DAT Quantitative Reasoning Practice Test 4

**1) Choice E is correct**

$g(x) = -2$, then $f(g(x)) = f(-2) = 3(-2)^3 + 5(-2)^2 + 2(-2) = -24 + 20 - 4 = -8$

**2) Choice E is correct**

Let $x$ be the width of the rectangle. Use Pythagorean Theorem:

$a^2 + b^2 = c^2$

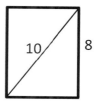

$x^2 + 8^2 = 10^2 \Rightarrow x^2 + 64 = 100 \Rightarrow x^2 = 100 - 64 = 36 \Rightarrow x = 6$

Perimeter of the rectangle = $2(length + width) = 2(8 + 6) = 2(14) = 28$

**3) Choice C is correct**

$x = \frac{1}{3}$ and $y = \frac{9}{21}$, substitute the values of $x$ and $y$ in the expression and simplify:

$\frac{1}{x} \div \frac{y}{3} \rightarrow \frac{1}{\frac{1}{3}} \div \frac{\frac{9}{21}}{3} \rightarrow \frac{1}{\frac{1}{3}} = 3$ and $\frac{\frac{9}{21}}{3} = \frac{9}{63} = \frac{1}{7}$. Then: $\frac{1}{\frac{1}{3}} \div \frac{\frac{9}{21}}{3} = 3 \div \frac{1}{7} = 3 \times 7 = 21$

**4) Choice A is correct**

$average\ (mean) = \frac{\text{sum of terms}}{\text{number of terms}} \Rightarrow 85 = \frac{\text{sum of terms}}{50} \Rightarrow sum = 85 \times 50 = 4250$

The difference of 94 and 69 is 25. Therefore, 25 should be subtracted from the sum.

$4250 - 25 = 4225, mean = \frac{\text{sum of terms}}{\text{number of terms}} \Rightarrow mean = \frac{4225}{50} = 84.5$

**5) Choice D is correct**

Solve for $x$. $x - 4 \leq 4x - 8 < 16 \Rightarrow$ (add 8 all sides) $-4 + 8 < 4x - 8 + 8 < 16 + 8 \Rightarrow$

$4 < 4x < 24 \Rightarrow$ (divide all sides by 4) $1 \leq x < 6$. $x$ is between 1 and 6. Choice D represents this inequality.

**6) Choice E is correct**

Use formula of rectangle prism volume.

$V = (length)(width)(height) \Rightarrow 2000 = (25)(10)(height) \Rightarrow height$
$= 2000 \div 250 = 8$

**7) Choice C is correct**

To find the number of possible outfit combinations, multiply number of options for each factor:

$3 \times 7 \times 4 = 84$

**8) Choice B is correct**

The diagonal of the square is 8. Let $x$ be the side. Use Pythagorean Theorem: $a^2 + b^2 = c^2$

$x^2 + x^2 = 8^2 \Rightarrow 2x^2 = 8^2 \Rightarrow 2x^2 = 64 \Rightarrow x^2 = 32 \Rightarrow x = \sqrt{32}$

The area of the square is: $\sqrt{32} \times \sqrt{32} = 32$

**9) Choice A is correct**

The width of the rectangle is twice its length. Let $x$ be the length. Then, $width = 2x$

Perimeter of the rectangle is $2\,(width + length) = 2(2x + x) = 60 \Rightarrow 6x = 60 \Rightarrow x = 10$

Length of the rectangle is 10 meters.

**10) Choice D is correct**

$average = \frac{\text{sum of terms}}{\text{number of terms}} \Rightarrow$ (average of 6 numbers) $12 = \frac{sum\ of\ numbers}{6} \Rightarrow$ sum of 6 numbers is $12 \times 6 = 72$,

(average of 4 numbers) $10 = \frac{sum\ of\ numbers}{4} \Rightarrow$ sum of 4 numbers is $10 \times 4 = 40$

$sum\ of\ 6\ numbers - sum\ of\ 4\ numbers = sum\ of\ 2\ numbers$

$72 - 40 = 32$, average of 2 numbers $= \frac{32}{2} = 16$

**11) Choice C is correct**

Solve for the sum of five numbers.

$average = \frac{\text{sum of terms}}{\text{number of terms}} \Rightarrow 24 = \frac{\text{sum of 5 numbers}}{5} \Rightarrow$ sum of 5 numbers $= 24 \times 5 = 120$

The sum of 5 numbers is 120. If a sixth number 42 is added, then the sum of 6 numbers is

$120 + 42 = 162$, $average = \frac{\text{sum of terms}}{\text{number of terms}} = \frac{162}{6} = 27$

**12) Choice D is correct**

Th ratio of boy to girls is $4: 7$. Therefore, there are 4 boys out of 11 students. To find the answer, first divide the total number of students by 11, then multiply the result by 4.

$66 \div 11 = 6 \Rightarrow 6 \times 4 = 24$, There are 24 boys and $42\ (66 - 24)$ girls. So, 18 more boys should be enrolled to make the ratio $1: 1$.

**13) Choice D is correct**

Jason needs an 76% average to pass for five exams. Therefore, the sum of 5 exams must be at lease $5 \times 76 = 380$, The sum of 4 exams is: $68 + 72 + 85 + 90 = 315$.

The minimum score Jason can earn on his fifth and final test to pass is:$380 - 315 = 65$

**14) Choice A is correct**

Let $x$ be the integer. Then: $2x - 5 = 53$. Add 5 both sides: $2x = 58$, Divide both sides by 2:

$x = 29$

**15) Choice B is correct**

Use simple interest formula:$I = prt$,($I$ = interest, p = principal, $r$ = rate, $t$ = time)

$I = (12000)(0.035)(2) = 840$

**16) Choice D is correct**

Simplify. $6x^2y^3(2x^2y)^3 = 6x^2y^3(8x^6y^3) = 48x^8y^6$

**17) Choice C is correct**

Surface Area of a cylinder $= 2\pi r(r + h)$, The radius of the cylinder is 6 inches and its height is 12 inches. $\pi$ is about 3.14. Then: Surface Area of a cylinder $= 2(\pi)(6)(6 + 12) = 216\,\pi = 678.24$

**18) Choice E is correct**

Use Pythagorean Theorem: $a^2 + b^2 = c^2$

$80^2 + 150^2 = c^2 \Rightarrow 6400 + 22500 = c^2 \Rightarrow 28900 = c^2 \Rightarrow c = 170$

**19) Choice E is correct**

Plug in 104 for $F$ and then solve for $C$.

$$C = \frac{5}{9}(F - 32) \Rightarrow C = \frac{5}{9}(140 - 32) \Rightarrow C = \frac{5}{9}(108) = 60$$

**20) Choice A is correct**

First, find the number. Let $x$ be the number. Write the equation and solve for $x$.

150% of a number is 75, then:$1.5 \times x = 75 \Rightarrow x = 75 \div 1.5 = 50$

95% of 50 is: $0.95 \times 50 = 47.5$

**21) Choice C is correct**

the population is increased by 15% and 20%. 15% increase changes the population to 115% of original population. For the second increase, multiply the result by 120%.

$(1.15) \times (1.20) = 1.38 = 138\%$.38 percent of the population is increased after two years.

**22) Choice C is correct**

Three times of 24,000 is 72,000. One sixth of them cancelled their tickets. One sixth of 72,000 equals 12,000 ($\frac{1}{6} \times 72000 = 12000$). 60,000 ($72000 - 12000 = 60000$) fans are attending this week.

**23) Choice E is correct**

The area of the square is 64 inches. Therefore, the side of the square is square root of the area.$\sqrt{64} = 8$ inches. Four times the side of the square is the perimeter:$4 \times 8 = 32\ inches$

**24) Choice D is correct**

The equation of a line is in the form of $y = mx + b$, where $m$ is the slope of the line and $b$ is the $y - intercept$ of the line. Two points (4,3) and (3,2) are on line A. Therefore, the slope of the line A is: $slope\ of\ line\ A = \frac{y_2 - y_1}{x_2 - x_1} = \frac{2-3}{3-4} = \frac{-1}{-1} = 1$

The slope of line A is 1. Thus, the formula of the line A is: $y = mx + b = x + b$, choose a point and plug in the values of $x$ and $y$ in the equation to solve for $b$. Let's choose point $(4, 3)$. Then:

$y = x + b \rightarrow 3 = 4 + b \rightarrow b = 3 - 4 = -1$

The equation of line A is: $y = x - 1$

Now, let's review the choices provided:

A. $(-1, 2)$        $y = x - 1 \rightarrow 2 = -1 - 1 = -2$      This is not true.

B. $(5, 7)$        $y = x - 1 \rightarrow 7 = 5 - 1 = 4$      This is not true.

C. $(3, 4)$        $y = x - 1 \rightarrow 4 = 3 - 1 = 2$      This is not true.

D. $(-1, -2)$        $y = x - 1 \rightarrow -2 = -1 - 1 = -2$      This is true!

E. $(-7, -9)$        $y = x - 1 \rightarrow -9 = -7 - 1 = -8$      This is not true!

**25) Choice E is correct**

$g(x) = -2$, then $f\big(g(x)\big) = f(-2) = 2\,(-2)^3 + 5(-2)^2 + 2(-2) = -16 + 20 - 4 = 0$

**26) Choice E is correct**

The formula for the area of the circle is: $A = \pi r^2$ .The area is $64\pi$. Therefore:$A = \pi r^2 \Rightarrow 64\pi = \pi r^2$

Divide both sides by $\pi$:$64 = r^2 \Rightarrow r = 8$. Diameter of a circle is $2 \times$ radius. Then:

Diameter $= 2 \times 8 = 16$

**27) Choice C is correct**

Write a proportion and solve for $x$.$\frac{3}{2} = \frac{x}{22} \Rightarrow 2x = 3 \times 22 \Rightarrow x = 33\ ft$

**28) Choice A is correct**

Use FOIL method. $(4x + 2y)(2x - y) = 8x^2 - 4xy + 4xy - 2y^2 = 8x^2 - 2y^2$

**29) Choice D is correct**

To solve absolute values equations, write two equations. $x - 10$ could be positive 3, or negative 3. Therefore, $x - 10 = 3 \Rightarrow x = 13, x - 10 = -3 \Rightarrow x = 7$, Find the product of solutions: $7 \times 13 = 91$

**30) Choice B is correct**

The equation of a line in slope intercept form is: $y = mx + b$. Solve for $y$. $4x - 2y = 8 \Rightarrow -2y = 8 - 4x \Rightarrow y = (8 - 4x) \div (-2) \Rightarrow y = 2x - 4$. The slope is 2. The slope of the line perpendicular to this line is: $m_1 \times m_2 = -1 \Rightarrow 2 \times m_2 = -1 \Rightarrow m_2 = -\frac{1}{2}$

**31) Choice C is correct**

Plug in the value of $x$ and $y$. $x = 3$ and $y = -2$,

$5(x - 2y) + (2 - x)^2 = 5(3 - 2(-2)) + (2 - 3)^2 = 5(3 + 4) + (-1)^2 = 35 + 1 = 36$

**32) Choice E is correct**

The distance between Jason and Joe is 15 miles. Jason running at 5.5 miles per hour and Joe is running at the speed of 7 miles per hour. Therefore, every hour the distance is 1.5 miles less.

$15 \div 1.5 = 10$

**33) Choice D is correct**

The failing rate is 11 out of 88 $= \frac{11}{88}$, Change the fraction to percent: $\frac{11}{88} \times 100\% = 12.5\%$

12.5 percent of students failed. Therefore, 87.5 percent of students passed the exam.

**34) Choice B is correct**

$$tan\theta = \frac{\text{opposite}}{\text{adjacent}}$$

$tan\theta = \frac{5}{12} \Rightarrow$ we have the following right triangle. Then:

$c = \sqrt{5^2 + 12^2} = \sqrt{25 + 144} = \sqrt{169} = 13$

$cos\theta = \frac{adjacent}{hypotenuse} = \frac{12}{13}$

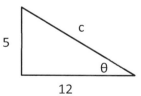

**35) Choice B is correct**

The area of trapezoid is: $\left(\frac{8+12}{2}\right) \times x = 100 \rightarrow 10x = 100 \rightarrow x = 10$

$$y = \sqrt{3^2 + 4^2} = 5$$

Perimeter is:   $12 + 10 + 8 + 5 = 35$

**36) Choice C is correct**

Set of number that are not composite between 1 and 25: $A = \{1, 2, 3, 5, 7, 11, 13, 17, 19, 23\}$

$$\text{Probability} = \frac{number\ of\ desired\ outcomes}{number\ of\ total\ outcomes} = \frac{10}{25} = \frac{2}{5}$$

**37) Choice D is correct**
   Check each choice provided:

A. 1    $\dfrac{4+5+8+11+}{5} = \dfrac{40}{5} = 8$

B. 4    $\dfrac{1+5+8+11+12}{5} = \dfrac{37}{5} = 7.4$

C. 5    $\dfrac{1+4+8+11+}{5} = \dfrac{36}{5} = 7.2$

D. 11    $\dfrac{1+4+5+8+1}{5} = \dfrac{30}{5} = 6$

E. 12    $\dfrac{1+4+5+8+11}{5} = \dfrac{29}{5} = 5.8$

**38) Choice A is correct**
$sinA = \frac{1}{3} \Rightarrow$

Since $sin\theta = \frac{opposite}{hypotenuse}$, we have the following right triangle. Then:

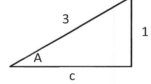

$$c = \sqrt{3^2 - 1^2} = \sqrt{9-1} = \sqrt{8}$$

$$cosA = \frac{\sqrt{8}}{3}$$

**39) Choice C is correct**
   Plug in the value of each choice in the inequality.

A. 1    $(1-2)^2 + 1 > 3(1) - 1 \rightarrow {}_2 > 2$    No!

B. 6    $(6-2)^2 + 1 > 3(6) - 1 \rightarrow {}_{17} > 17$    No!

C. 8    $(8-2)^2 + 1 > 3(8) - 1 \rightarrow {}_{37} > 23$    Bingo!

D. 3    $(3-2)^2 + 1 > 3(3) - 1 \rightarrow {}_2 > 8$    No!

E.  4        $(4 - 2)^2 + 1 > 3(4) - 1 \rightarrow 5 > 11$        No!

**40) Choice A is correct.**

The relationship among all sides of right triangle $30° - 60° - 90°$ is provided in the following triangle: Sine of 30° equals to: $\frac{opposite}{hypotenuse} = \frac{x}{2x} = \frac{1}{2}$

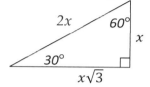

## DAT Quantitative Reasoning Practice Test 5

**1) Choice C is correct**

Plug in the value of $x$ and $y$: $x = 2$ and $y = -1$

$2(2x - y) + (4 - x)^2 = x^2 - 4x - 2y + 16 = (2)^2 - 4(2) - 2(-1) + 16 = 14$

**2) Choice E is correct**

Use formula of rectangle prism volume : $V = (length)(width)(height) \Rightarrow 1,500 = (15)(10)(height) \Rightarrow height = 1,500 \div 150 = 10$

**3) Choice C is correct**

To find the number of possible outfit combinations, multiply number of options for each factor: $5 \times 4 \times 3 = 60$

**4) Choice E is correct**

$g(x) = 3$, then $f\big(g(x)\big) = f(3) = (3)^3 - 2(3)^2 + 8(3) = 27 - 18 + 24 = 33$

**5) Choice E is correct**

Let $x$ be the width of the rectangle. Use Pythagorean Theorem:

$a^2 + b^2 = c^2$

$x^2 + 8^2 = 10^2 \Rightarrow x^2 + 64 = 100 \Rightarrow x^2 = 100 - 64 = 36 \Rightarrow x = 6$

Perimeter of the rectangle $= 2(length + width) = 2(8 + 6) = 2(14) = 28$

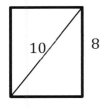

**6) Choice B is correct**

The perimeter of the trapezoid is 42. Therefore, the missing side (height) is $= 42 - 9 - 16 - 12 = 5$ , Area of a trapezoid: $A = \frac{1}{2}h(b_1 + b_2) = \frac{1}{2}(5)(9 + 12) = 52.5$

**7) Choice C is correct**

Solve for the sum of seven numbers: $average = \frac{sum\ of\ terms}{number\ of\ terms} \Rightarrow 32 = \frac{sum\ of\ 7\ numbers}{7} \Rightarrow$
$sum\ of\ 7\ numbers = 32 \times 7 = 224$, The sum of 7 numbers is 224. If a eighth number 18 is added, then the sum of 8 numbers is :

$224 + 18 = 242$ , $average = \frac{sum\ of\ terms}{number\ of\ terms} = \frac{242}{8} = 30.25$

**8) Choice C is correct**

Th ratio of boy to girls is $4: 7$. Therefore, there are 4 boys out of 11 students. To find the answer, first divide the total number of students by 11, then multiply the result by 4.

$44 \div 11 = 4 \Rightarrow 4 \times 4 = 16$ , There are 16 boys and $28(44 - 16)$ girls. So, 12 more boys should be enrolled to make the ratio $1: 1$

**9) Choice D is correct**

Isolate and solve for $x$: $\frac{2}{3}x + \frac{1}{6} = \frac{1}{3} \Rightarrow \frac{2}{3}x = \frac{1}{3} - \frac{1}{6} = \frac{1}{6} \Rightarrow \frac{2}{3}x = \frac{1}{6}$

Multiply both sides by the reciprocal of the coefficient of $x$.

$(\frac{3}{2})\frac{2}{3}x = \frac{1}{6}(\frac{3}{2}) \Rightarrow x = \frac{3}{12} = \frac{1}{4}$

**10) Choice B is correct**

Use simple interest formula: $I = prt$, $(I = interest, p = principal, r = rate, t = time)$

$I = (16,000)(0.025)(3) = 1,200$

**11) Choice E is correct**

Jason needs an 75% average to pass for five exams. Therefore, the sum of 5 exams must be at lease $5 \times 75 = 375$, The sum of 4 exams is: $68 + 72 + 85 + 90 = 315$.

The minimum score Jason can earn on his fifth and final test to pass is: $375 - 315 = 60$

**12) Choice D is correct**

To get a sum of 6 for two dice, we can get 5 different options: $(5,1), (4,2), (3,3), (2,4), (1,5)$

To get a sum of 9 for two dice, we can get 4 different options: $(6,3), (5,4), (4,5), (3,6)$

Therefore, there are 9 options to get the sum of 6 or 9. Since, we have $6 \times 6 = 36$ total options, the probability of getting a sum of 6 and 9 is 9 out of 36 or $\frac{1}{4}$.

**13) Choice C is correct**

Surface Area of a cylinder $= 2\pi r(r + h)$, The radius of the cylinder is $3(6 \div 2)$ inches and its height is 8 inches. Therefore, Surface Area of a cylinder $= 2\pi(3)(3 + 8) = 66\pi$

**14) Choice D is correct**

Use FOIL method: $(3x - y)(2x + 2y) = 6x^2 + 6xy - 2xy - 2y^2 = 6x^2 + 4xy - 2y^2$

**15) Choice D is correct**

To solve absolute values equations, write two equations. $x - 12$ could be positive 4, or negative $-4$. Therefore, $x - 12 = 4 \Rightarrow x = 16$, $x - 12 = -4 \Rightarrow x = 8$ . Find the product of solutions: $8 \times 16 = 128$

**16) Choice B is correct**

The equation of a line in slope intercept form is: $y = mx + b$

Solve for $y$: $4x - 2y = 12 \Rightarrow -2y = 12 - 4x \Rightarrow y = (12 - 4x) \div (-2) \Rightarrow$

$y = 2x - 6$, The slope is 2, The slope of the line perpendicular to this line is:

$m_1 \times m_2 = -1 \Rightarrow 2 \times m_2 = -1 \Rightarrow m_2 = -\frac{1}{2}$

**17) Choice C is correct**

Three times of 18,000 is 54,000. One sixth of them cancelled their tickets.

One sixth of 54,000 equals 9,000 ($\frac{1}{6} \times 54,000 = 9,000$).

45,000 ($54,000 - 9,000 = 45,000$) fans are attending this week.

### 18) Choice E is correct

The area of the square is 81 inches. Therefore, the side of the square is square root of the area. $\sqrt{81} = 9$ inches. Four times the side of the square is the perimeter: $4 \times 9 = 36 \ inches$

### 19) Choice E is correct

First factor the function: $(x - 4)(x - 3)$. To find the zeros, $f(x)$ should be zero: $f(x) = (x - 4)(x - 3) = 0$, Therefore, the zeros are, $(x - 4) = 0 \Rightarrow x = 4, (x - 3) = 0 \Rightarrow x = 3$

### 20) Choice C is correct

$$average \ (mean) = \frac{sum \ of \ terms}{number \ of \ terms} \Rightarrow 88 = \frac{sum \ of \ terms}{50} \Rightarrow sum = 88 \times 50 = 4400$$

The difference of 94 and 69 is 25. Therefore, 25 should be subtracted from the sum.

$4400 - 25 = 4375$, $mean = \frac{sum \ of \ terms}{number \ of \ terms} \Rightarrow mean = \frac{4375}{50} = 87.5$

### 21) Choice B is correct

Plug in 122 for $F$ and then solve for $C$.

$$C = \frac{5}{9} (F - 32) \Rightarrow C = \frac{5}{9} (122 - 32) \Rightarrow C = \frac{5}{9} (90) = 50$$

### 22) Choice A is correct

The width of the rectangle is twice its length. Let $x$ be the length. Then, $width = 2x$

Perimeter of the rectangle is: $2 \ (width + length) = 2(2x + x) = 120 \Rightarrow 6x = 120 \Rightarrow x = 20$. Length of the rectangle is 20 meters.

### 23) Choice A is correct

First, find the number. Let $x$ be the number. Write the equation and solve for $x$.

150% of a number is 75, then: $1.5 \times x = 75 \Rightarrow x = 75 \div 1.5 = 50$. 90% of 50 is: $0.9 \times 50 = 45$

### 24) Choice E is correct

Solve for $y$: $8x - 4y = 8$, Divided both sides by $-4$: $\frac{8}{-4} x - \frac{4}{-4} y = \frac{8}{-4}$

$-2x + y = -2 \rightarrow y = 2x - 2$, Then: The slope of the line is 2.

### 25) Choice C is correct

The population is increased by 12% and 25%. 12% increase changes the population to 112% of original population. For the second increase, multiply the result by 125%: $(1.12) \times (1.25) = 1.40 = 140\%$, 40 percent of the population is increased after two years.

### 26) Choice D is correct

$average = \frac{sum\ of\ terms}{number\ of\ terms} \Rightarrow$ (average of 8 numbers) $14 = \frac{sum\ of\ numbers}{8} \Rightarrow$ sum of 8 numbers is: $14 \times 8 = 112$

(average of 6 numbers) $12 = \frac{sum\ of\ numbers}{6} \Rightarrow$ sum of 6 numbers is: $12 \times 6 = 72$

$sum\ of\ 8\ numbers - sum\ of\ 6\ numbers = sum\ of\ 2\ numbers$

$112 - 72 = 40 \qquad$ average of 2 numbers $= \frac{40}{2} = 20$

### 27) Choice E is correct

Five years ago, Amy was three times as old as Mike. Mike is 10 years now. Therefore, 5 years ago Mike was 5 years. Five years ago, Amy was: $A = 3 \times 5 = 15$ , Now Amy is 20 years old: $15 + 5 = 20$

### 28) Choice C is correct

Write a proportion and solve for $x$: $\frac{4}{3} = \frac{x}{18} \Rightarrow 3x = 18 \times 4 \Rightarrow x = \frac{72}{3} = 24\ ft$

### 29) Choice A is correct.

Let the number be $A$. Then: $x = y\% \times A$. Solve for $A$. $x = \frac{y}{100} \times A$

Multiply both sides by $\frac{100}{y}$: $x \times \frac{100}{y} = \frac{y}{100} \times \frac{100}{y} \times A \rightarrow A = \frac{100x}{y}$

### 30) Choice C is correct

$tangent\ \beta = \dfrac{1}{cotangent\ \beta} = \dfrac{1}{1} = 1$

### 31) Choice A is correct

One liter $= 1000\ cm^3 \rightarrow 6$ liters $= 6000\ cm^3$

$6000 = 15 \times 5 \times h \rightarrow h = \frac{6000}{75} = 80\ cm$

### 32) Choice B is correct

$\frac{2}{3} \times 90 = 60$

### 33) Choice C is correct

I. $|a| < 1 \rightarrow -1 < a < 1$

Multiply all sides by $b$. Since, $b > 0 \rightarrow -b < ba < b$ (it is true!)

II. Since, $-1 < a < 1, and\ a < 0 \rightarrow -a > a^2 > a$ (plug in $-\frac{1}{2}$, and check!) (It's false)

III. $-1 < a < 1$, *multiply all sides by* 2, *then:* $-2 < 2a < 2$

Subtract 3 from all sides. Then: $-2 - 3 < 2a - 3 < 2 - 3 \rightarrow -5 < 2a - 3 < -1$ (It is true!)

**34) Choice E is correct**

Use Pythagorean Theorem: $a^2 + b^2 = c^2$

$80^2 + 150^2 = c^2 \Rightarrow 6400 + 22500 = c^2 \Rightarrow 28900 = c^2 \Rightarrow c = 170$

**35) Choice C is correct**

Let $x$ be the number. Write the equation and solve for $x$.

$30\% \ of \ x = 12 \Rightarrow 0.30x = 12 \Rightarrow x = 12 \div 0.30 = 40$

**36) Choice C is correct**

The distance between Jason and Joe is 15 miles. Jason running at 4.5 miles per hour and Joe is running at the speed of 7 miles per hour. Therefore, every hour the distance is 2.5 miles less. $15 \div 2.5 = 6$

**37) Choice D is correct**

The failing rate is 11 out of $55 = \frac{11}{55}$, Change the fraction to percent: $\frac{11}{55} \times 100\% = 20\%$

20 percent of students failed. Therefore, 80 percent of students passed the exam.

**38) Choice D is correct**

A. $f(x) = x^2 - 5$      if     $x = 1 \rightarrow f(1) = (1)^2 - 5 = 1 - 5 = -4 \neq 5$

B. $f(x) = x^2 - 1$      if     $x = 1 \rightarrow f(1) = (1)^2 - 1 = 1 - 1 = 0 \neq 5$

C. $f(x) = \sqrt{x + 2}$      if     $x = 1 \rightarrow f(1) = \sqrt{1 + 2} = \sqrt{3} \neq 5$

D. $f(x) = \sqrt{x} + 4$      if     $x = 1 \rightarrow f(1) = \sqrt{1} + 4 = 5$

E. $f(x) = \sqrt{x + 1} + 4$      if     $x = 1 \rightarrow f(1) = \sqrt{1 + 1} + 4 \neq 5$

**39) Choice B is correct**

Plug in $z/3$ for $z$ and simplify.

$$x_1 = \frac{8y + \dfrac{r}{r+1}}{\dfrac{z}{3}} = \frac{8y + \dfrac{r}{r+1}}{\dfrac{3 \times 6}{z}} = \frac{8y + \dfrac{r}{r+1}}{3 \times \dfrac{6}{z}} = \frac{1}{3} \times \frac{8y + \dfrac{r}{r+1}}{\dfrac{6}{z}} = \frac{x}{3}$$

**40) Choice C is correct**

Substitute $x$ by 6 and $y$ by 28 in the equation. Then:

$6 \blacksquare 28 = \sqrt{6^2 + 28} = \sqrt{36 + 28} = \sqrt{64} = 8$

## "Effortless Math Education" Publications

Effortless Math authors' team strives to prepare and publish the best quality DAT Quantitative Reasoning learning resources to make learning Math easier for all. We hope that our publications help you learn Math in an effective way and prepare for the DAT test.

We all in Effortless Math wish you good luck and successful studies!

Effortless Math Authors

# www.EffortlessMath.com

... So Much More Online!

✓ FREE Math lessons

✓ More Math learning books!

✓ Mathematics Worksheets

✓ Online Math Tutors

**Need a PDF version of this book?**

Visit www.EffortlessMath.com